The Hospital for Special Surgery Rheumatoid Arthritis Handbook

STEPHEN A. PAGET, M.D.,
MICHAEL D. LOCKSHIN, M.D.,
AND SUZANNE LOEBL

John Wiley & Sons, Inc.

S

*D*edicated to the memory of Emmanuel Rudd, M.D.
St. Petersburg, 1914 — New York, 1995

*Who spent his professional life
at the Hospital for Special Surgery,
a friend of every arthritis patient
fortunate enough to cross his path...
and for David always*

Published by John Wiley & Sons, Inc.

Published simultaneously in Canada

No part of this publication may be reproduced, stored in a retrieval system, or transmitted in
any form or by any means, electronic, mechanical, photocopying, recording, scanning, or
otherwise, except as permitted under Section 107 or 108 of the 1976 United States Copyright
Act, without either the prior written permission of the Publisher, or authorization through
payment of the appropriate per-copy fee to the Copyright Clearance Center, 222 Rosewood
Drive, Danvers, MA 01923, (978) 750-8400, fax (978) 750-4744. Requests to the Publisher for
permission should be addressed to the Permissions Department, John Wiley & Sons, Inc., 605
Third Avenue, New York, NY 10158-0012, (212) 850-6011, fax (212) 850-6008, email:
PERMREQ@WILEY.COM.

This publication is designed to provide accurate and authoritative information in regard to
the subject matter covered. It is sold with the understanding that the publisher is not
engaged in rendering professional services. If professional advice or other expert assistance
is required, the services of a competent professional person should be sought.

Library of Congress Cataloging-in-Publication Data has been applied for.

ISBN 0-471-41045-4

Printed in the United States of America
10 9 8 7 6 5 4 3 2 1

Contents

Acknowledgments

—◆—

The Hospital for Special Surgery Rheumatoid Arthritis Handbook reflects the skill and knowledge of many experts. Special thanks are due to key staff members as follows, in alphabetical order:

Adina Batterman, CSW, program coordinator for the HSS Rheumatoid Arthritis Education and Support Group (Chapter 14)

Laura Broach, PT (Chapter 19)

Todd Cronin, PT, who is an expert at getting people with arthritis moving (Chapter 12)

Glen Garrison, CPO, Cped, Director (Chapter 19)

Suzanne Graziano, RN, MS, ONC, CAN, clinical nurse specialist, Department of Nursing Administration (Chapters 16, 17, and 18)

Annabel Griffith, OTR (Chapters 13 and 19)

Roberta Horton, ACSW, Program and Research Coordinator, HSS Department of Patient Care (Chapter 14)

Bryan Nestor, M.D., assistant attending orthopaedic surgeon (Chapters 17 and 18)

Thomas P. Sculco, M.D., director of orthopaedic surgery and chief of the Surgical Arthritis Service (Chapter 16)

Medical self-help books draw on works written by others. The authors consulted numerous textbooks, journals, scientific reports, and patient education publications, and attended relevant scientific meetings.

Specific thanks are due to the Arthritis Foundation for their excellent publications and to the American College of Rheumatology and the Association for Rheumatology Health Professionals for their *Primer on Rheumatic Diseases* and their excellent scientific meetings. Particular thanks are due to Marian A. Minor, Ph.D., PT, for providing information on how patients with rheumatoid arthritis can exercise.

This handbook is richly illustrated. Thanks are due to Lippincott, Williams & Wilkins for permission to use the exercises presented in Chapter 12, published in *The Manual of Rheumatology and Outpatient Orthopedic Disorders,* by Stephen Paget, Paul Pellicci, and John F. Beary. Exercises provided in the chapters dealing with total hip and knee replacement, as well as other illustrations related to surgery and the protection of newly implanted joints, are provided courtesy of Suzanne Graziano, Department of Nursing Administration, Hospital for Special Surgery. The anatomical drawings are from the *Columbia-Presbyterian Osteoarthritis Handbook,* edited by Ronald P. Grelsamer and Suzanne Loebl, and are courtesy of Hungry Mind Publishers. We also want to thank Amgen, Inc. for the drawing of an inflamed joint; Wright Medical Technology, Arlington, TN, for the photographs of the total knee, total hip, and Swanson finger joint implants; Dr. Alfred R. Swanson for the photographs of the hands before and after surgery; Annabel Griffith for the photograph of the dynamic hand splint; and Glenn Garrison for the foot exercises. Thanks are due to the staff of HSS operating rooms, who provided information when necessary as the authors watched the actual joint replacement surgery, and Suzanne Graziano, who checked the surgery chapters for accuracy.

The authors appreciate the help of their colleagues. Any mistaken interpretation, however, is solely their responsibility.

We want to thank Chip Rossetti, our editor at Wiley, for shepherding this book through its editing and production process.

To be effective, self-help books rely on relating actual experiences. An immense debt of gratitude is owed to the patients who shared their experiences with the authors. Their names have been changed, but their actual words and feelings are used throughout the book.

Introduction

WHO SHOULD READ THIS BOOK

This book is written for people who suffer from rheumatoid arthritis as well as for their families and friends. Rheumatoid arthritis (RA) is a chronic disease for which self-care is crucial. The more you know about the disease, the better you will be able to cope with it. However, in no way can your knowledge substitute for the care provided by your physician and other members of your health team. This handbook's purpose is to amplify and reinforce their instructions and help you participate more fully in your treatment.

WHY THIS BOOK

For a very long time, rheumatoid arthritis was a mystery. Paradoxically, its symptoms are characteristic of arthritis, a disorder most commonly seen among the elderly—yet, in this case, they occur in the young and vigorous. It is a disorder associated with pain, weight loss, and eventually joint deformity. It is a malady that resembles an infection, yet for years it yielded no identifiable "bug." Gradually, the mystery and helplessness lifted. About 150 years ago, it was shown that a new drug, aspirin—whose discovery itself was based on a folk remedy—offered temporary relief. Another drug—gold—was stumbled upon during the 1920s. At long last, on the eve of World War II, scientists realized that rheumatoid arthritis was associated with a malfunction of the immune system. Researchers were finally on the right track. The immune system, however, was a mystery of its own, and even today its function is still being unraveled. Fortunately, enough is known to make your rheumatoid arthritis treatable.

It is absolutely essential to minimize the damage that rheumatoid arthritis can inflict on your body, but keeping the disease in check can be a major undertaking. Helping you to do so is the lifework of the authors of this book.

How This Book Is Organized

Chapters 1 through 5 explore the physiological processes that malfunction due to RA and the manner in which these irregularities affect the body. Readers learn about joints, body mechanics, and the immune system, and become familiar with the language used to describe various aspects of the disease, its diagnosis, and treatment.

Chapters 6 through 9 are devoted to drug therapy, one of the principal avenues for better treatment. In addition to general information about medication, the chapters review the different classes of drugs used to treat RA—analgesics, anti-inflammatory agents, immunosuppressants, and corticosteroids—and explore their similarities and differences. Special sections deal with questions you need to ask about newly prescribed drugs: potential side effects, how long to take a specific medication, why it works, and other details.

Chapter 10 explores specific considerations of having a baby when suffering from RA.

Chapters 11, 12, and 13 review nondrug aspects of treatment: nutrition and physical and occupational therapy. Sound nutrition plays a role in the well-being of people suffering from rheumatoid arthritis. Certain drugs, especially corticosteroids, have a major impact on metabolism and body weight and may require a modification of your food intake. Chapter 11 makes specific suggestions on how to handle some of these issues, and also discusses vitamins and popular supplements such as glucosamine and evening primrose oil. Chapter 12 reviews both recreational and therapeutic exercises. Specific exercises designed to keep the body limber and in good shape are suggested. Dysfunctional joints, especially those of the hands, may make activities of daily living (performing routine tasks) difficult. Chapter 13 outlines how to minimize and/or solve these problems, and how to rehabilitate small joints.

In Chapter 14 we meet a group of patients with RA and explore the psychological impact of this chronic disease. Courage and self-reliance are as much a hallmark of those affected by RA as rheumatoid factor or genetic predisposition. We explore ways of coping with difficult aspects of RA, especially the unpredictability of the disease. Strategies are offered on how to manage your sex life and on how to deal with depression and pain.

Remarkable Jerry Walsh is the subject of Chapter 15. He developed the disease at age 18. Eventually, he became a patient at the Mayo Clinic in Rochester, Minnesota, and was able to profit from the remarkable advances in the treatment of RA that occurred during the second half of the 20th century. Jerry was at Mayo soon after the discovery of the almost miraculous effects of the corticosteroids and walked out of the hospital with the assistance of two crutches. Toward the end of his life, he underwent a double hip replacement at the Mayo Clinic. Jerry's courage and determination are an inspiration to all suffering from chronic disease.

Chapters 16 through 19 explore the surgical options available to patients suffering from RA. The very detailed information about commonly used surgical procedures may help you in the inevitable decision-making process that precedes surgery. Knowing what to expect before, during, and after the operation may lessen the anxiety that accompanies all major medical interventions.

A glossary and a set of frequently asked questions and their answers complete the book.

YOUR MEDICAL TEAM

Founded in 1899, the Hospital for Special Surgery (HSS) is one of the nation's oldest and best orthopedic hospitals. From early on, rheumatoid arthritis has been one of its special concerns. The following experts, all on the hospital staff, have provided information that may further your understanding of rheumatoid arthritis and its management. The information provided is designed to amplify your knowledge. At no time should it replace the instructions provided by your physician or any other member of your own health care provider.

Drs. Stephen Paget and Michael Lockshin provide general information about RA, as well as about standard drug therapy. Both have devoted their entire professional lives to the treatment of rheumatoid arthritis and other autoimmune disorders. Todd Cronin, a physical therapist, is an expert at getting people with RA back on their feet. Annabel Griffith, an occupational therapist, specializes in therapy of the hands. Adina Batterman and Roberta Horton are social workers who help people cope with the emotional aspects of dealing with a painful, chronic disorder. Suzanne Graziano, a registered nurse, lets you participate in the presurgical courses that she created for patients about to undergo total joint-replacement surgery. Drs. Thomas P. Sculco and Bryan Nestor provide in-depth information on hip and knee replacement, and even let you peek into the operating room. Last, but not least, Laura Broach and Glen Garrison provide exercises for your feet and help you pick well-fitting, comfortable shoes.

How to Use This Book

"We have nothing to fear but fear itself," said Franklin Delano Roosevelt, himself the target of a crippling disease, when America had to emerge from its Great Depression during the 1930s. Rheumatoid arthritis is a scary disease—but with knowledge, good medical care, and a bit of luck, you will be able to lead a normal, fruitful existence. The authors have done their best to demystify the disease and the medical jargon that is often used in health care.

In addition to in-depth information, this handbook provides as much practical information as the authors could muster. Since most people are encouraged by the experiences of others coping with similar disorders, the authors have included the stories of fellow sufferers. Chapter 1 deals with five patients who have longstanding RA. Since these interviews one of them has given birth to a healthy baby. In Chapter 2, we share the experience of Henry S. as he discovers that he suffers from an aggressive case of RA.

We hope that *The Hospital for Special Surgery Rheumatoid Arthritis Handbook* will become your trusted friend. Use it to review scientific information, to look up information about particular topics, and perhaps even to derive comfort from those who are successfully living with rheumatoid arthritis.

1

The Empowered Patient

══➤◄((❁))►◄══

This chapter relates how five individuals struggle with their rheumatoid arthritis.

THE BIRTH OF VENUS

Ever since 1477 when Sandro Botticelli painted her, 16-year old Simonetta Vespucci has mesmerized the crowd that comes to pay homage. She stands on an immense scallop shell. Her amber eyes gaze into the distance. She dreams. Strands of red hair cascade down her back, waft in the wind, and ineffectively shield her voluptuous body. She is Venus, the goddess of love and beauty. Sandro Botticelli painted her as she emerged fully grown from the depths of the blue Mediterranean.

The real-life Simonetta might not have felt as serene as she looks. Doctors have examined the figure's slightly deformed fingers, the sausage-like enlargement of her left index finger, and her swollen ankles and believe that the world's most beautiful woman suffered from rheumatoid arthritis. The young lady died of tuberculosis soon after Botticelli depicted her in this and two other canvasses. All three were painted to celebrate a major Florentine festival.

It took half a millennium before the nature of Simonetta Vespucci's disease was clearly identified. Both *rheumatism* and *arthritis* are old terms. In *The Merry Wives of Windsor*, Shakespeare talks of a "raw, rheumatic day," because even then arthritis and rheumatism were associated with

5

damp weather. During the 16th century, the French physician Guillaume was the first to associate the word *rheumatism* with joint ailments.

For centuries, doctors lumped all disorders involving joint pain together. Thomas Sydenham (1624–1689), one of medicine's great investigators, began sorting out the mix and provided an accurate clinical description of what might have been rheumatoid arthritis. The term *rheumatoid arthritis* was coined by A. B. Garrod, another English physician, in 1858.

Medical X rays, which made their debut in 1895, enabled physicians to actually look at hard structures such as bones and joint tissues and see the damage arthritis wrought in their patients. The belief that rheumatoid arthritis is the consequence of some bacterial infection was prevalent at the beginning of the 20th century. It serendipitously led to the discovery of several useful treatments, most notably gold and drugs used to treat malaria.

In 1940, the rheumatoid factor that is present in most patients suffering from rheumatoid arthritis was simultaneously discovered in Norway and at Columbia Presbyterian Medical Center in New York. By then, physicians were aware of the inflammatory nature of rheumatoid arthritis. In 1940, Bernard Comroe, an American physician, coined the term *rheumatologist* to designate an arthritis specialist.

It is understandable that the great variability of the disease's presentation and course, together with its fortunate, albeit rare, ability to go into remission, made it difficult to recognize its nature. Even today, rheumatologists are uncertain about the course the disease might follow in any particular patient.

Like most chronic disorders, rheumatoid arthritis is ideally suited for self-care. Its management involves a variety of facets. Before embarking on a review of these aspects of care, we shall visit with five patients who, like Botticelli's Venus, lead full, satisfying lives in spite of serious rheumatoid arthritis. Details of their treatment are in later chapters of this book.

MARION I.[1]

Marion I. storms up Broadway on her way to lunch. A graduate of Cornell's Hotel School, Marion is now an executive at Delta Airlines. She is in

---

[1]Except for Venus, everybody in this chapter is real and facts are based on interviews. To protect privacy, names and certain characteristics have been changed.

charge of arranging hotel accommodations for the company's ever-expanding, all-inclusive vacation tours. Marion just returned from the West Coast and is about to travel to Europe for a meeting with other top-level executives. "Jet lag does not affect me," she says in an offhanded manner.

Sports—swimming, skiing, hiking—were always important in her family. When time did not permit her to plan activities, Marion jogged regularly. Twelve years ago, she was working as a hotel consultant in Los Angeles. Most mornings, she raced up and down that city's steep hills. One day she injured her knee. She was 26 years old.

"I had torn my meniscus and needed arthroscopic surgery," she recalls. An arthroscope is a small fiber-optic surgical instrument used for diagnosis and minor joint surgery. The procedure usually does not require hospitalization, and patients are up and about within a few days.

After the surgery, Marion recalls, her knee did not heal. "When the physician investigated, he discovered that my sedimentation rate was sky-high."

A few more tests confirmed that Marion had rheumatoid arthritis. She was in pain, especially at night. "I was terribly stiff—so stiff that I could not even lift my blanket. My feet hurt; my fingers and elbows were excruciatingly painful. The doctors ordered splints to prevent my wrists and hands from becoming deformed and prescribed aspirin, Feldene, and other stuff to reduce the inflammation. Nobody had told me that I had to take these drugs with food, so my stomach revolted.

"I discovered that I was feeling better as long as I moved about. So when I got a bit better, I quit my desk job. During the next 6 months, I just traveled. Then my money ran out."

Marion moved to Canada, found a new job, and became a patient of Dr. Smith, a world-renowned rheumatologist. Her doctor decided to try gold shots. Gold, derived from the precious metal, has been used successfully for selected rheumatoid arthritis patients since the 1920s. In approximately one-third of cases, gold appears to cure arthritis. Actually, certain drugs induce a remission, which means that the rheumatoid arthritis is present but its symptoms are dormant.

Marion developed a severe allergic reaction to the specific gold preparation Dr. Smith used. Fortunately, doctor and patient persevered. Another gold preparation worked, and Marion went into remission. This was 10 years ago, and she has been fine ever since. She is still conscientiously taking a gold shot every 5 weeks. From time to time, she and her physician discuss discontinuing the gold, but they never quite dare. "What if the rheumatoid arthritis comes back?" Marion wonders.

Even though Marion only had active rheumatoid arthritis for 2 years, her body exhibits its ravages:

"My feet are all crippled," she says. "I have hammer toes. The tendons in my feet have shifted, and my elbow is very weak.

"I try to protect my body as best I can, and do exercises and sports in moderation. I am extremely careful not to overdo things. I try to ignore my rheumatoid arthritis, and when friends ask whether I am depressed because I have RA, I tell them that compared to other chronic disorders, RA is not that bad."

"My daughter refuses to be defeated," Marion's Chicago-based father says. "We are grateful that the gold worked. Still, it was a terrible shock when we learned that our child was suffering from a chronic, potentially crippling disease. With hindsight I regret that I did not hop onto a plane when she became sick and that she had to handle her acute illness by herself." He, however, hopes that he will never have to put his "hindsight" to the test.

JANE M.

"I can't talk today," Jane M., the editor of the *Rockland News,* says. "I am off skiing—the first time in 2 years."

Six years earlier, as Jane got out of bed, her feet felt incredibly stiff. She limped downstairs and went to work. A few weeks later, her knees felt stiff. Then it was her hands. By Christmas, she could no longer hold a pencil.

"The pain just flew around my body," Jane recalled. "I was turning into the Tin Man."

Jane went to her primary care physician at her small local hospital, who prescribed Voltaren, one of the newer nonsteroidal anti-inflammatory drugs (NSAIDs). She also talked to her father, a board-certified rheumatologist. Both physicians suspected that she suffered from rheumatoid arthritis.

That spring, Jane and a friend were to tour China. "I flew to the West Coast, and when I emerged from the plane after the long and painful ride, my friend was shocked. In spite of the incredible stiffness, I carried on and had a wonderful time."

When Jane got back home, she had a proper diagnostic workup. She did have rheumatoid arthritis, got a shot of cortisone, and eventually took methotrexate.

"I went into remission. But I don't trust methotrexate, and after a year I tapered it off. I was well for 2 years, but then my rheumatoid arthritis came back. Now I am back on methotrexate and I am doing better. I am scared of methotrexate and don't take my full dose of it, but I am increasing it slowly. I expect to be fine."

REVEREND B.

Methotrexate also made a big difference to Reverend B., the retired rector of Grace Church in Brooklyn. Eighteen years ago, when he was 50, he had trouble walking and "felt stiff all over."

The reverend's mother had suffered from rheumatoid arthritis, so he guessed that he, too, had the same disease. A few tests confirmed his self-diagnosis. It did not upset him, since his mother lived to be 87.

Reverend B. had easy access to excellent therapy in New York. He started taking aspirin, followed by Indocin, an older NSAID. Both medications upset his stomach. Then his physician suggested gold injections. After a few rough months, during which he also received corticosteroids and therapeutic exercises, his rheumatoid arthritis subsided.

Reverend B. served his church for 26 years. Three years ago, he retired and moved to his grandfather's old summer place in Vermont. "It is great living here," he said. "I have known this place all my life and it is like coming back home."

To keep in shape, Reverend B. walks a couple of miles each day. He has not quite given up the pulpit. He serves as a guest minister at various congregations throughout New Hampshire. Even though his disease had responded to gold, his New Hampshire rheumatologist switched him to methotrexate. "It is a wonderful pill," Reverend B. says. "Much better than gold. Instead of those endless injections, a weekly pill does the trick."

The rheumatoid arthritis, however, has left its marks. The reverend's fingers are deformed and cannot wield a tennis racquet. He has trouble with small hand movements and recently he underwent hand surgery that improved function.

Still, he is grateful and advises his fellow sufferers to find a good doctor, follow medical advice, and do as much exercise as possible.

SAMANTHA F.

Not everybody with rheumatoid arthritis does as well as Reverend B., Jane M., and Marion I. Samantha is a lawyer, working for a large multinational corporate firm. Her office is in downtown New York. Whenever she can, she takes cabs to work. When her arthritis is extremely bad, she works from home. Samantha is in charge of the firm's shipping contracts, and she works with phones and computers. Her smiling face, sparkling blue eyes, and relaxed expression are a pleasure to behold. Her features also belie the fact that excruciating pain has dominated her for 20 years.

"Nobody believes the amounts of the narcotics oxycodone, Demerol, and morphine that I require when I am in extreme pain," she explains. "As a matter of fact, I have a letter from my doctor which reassures unfamiliar physicians that it is all right to prescribe such large doses," she says.

Illness, no matter how severe, has always been only one part of Samantha's life. She has always worked. She raised her son, Charlie, as a single mother, and now lives on her own.

"I had my first rheumatic flare when I was 30 and was 3 months pregnant," Samantha recalled. "This in itself is unusual. Rheumatoid arthritis usually vanishes during pregnancy. At first, I did not pay much attention to my discomfort. I took my bar exam when I was 5 months pregnant. At the time, my two thumbs were killing me. I simply splinted them to cocktail forks. That relieved the pain. I passed the bar, gave birth, and stayed home until Charlie was 1 year old.

"By then I knew I had some form of rheumatoid or inflammatory arthritis. My husband left, I went back to work, and Charlie and I carried on as best we could."

From the beginning, Samantha took charge of her illness. She is an expert at self-care. Her freezer is full of gel packs, and her kitchen drawers are loaded with various splints. Samantha owns a TENS (transcutaneous electric nerve stimulation) machine. (The instrument delivers low-intensity electric impulses that relieve pain by an unknown mechanism.) She is knowledgeable about antiarthritis drugs. Over the years, she has taken all of them: aspirin—"until I developed an ulcer"—most of the 20-odd nonsteroidal anti-inflammatory drugs as soon as they were approved by the FDA, gold, penicillamine, and, of course, corticosteroids (see Chapters 7, 8, and 9). "You name it, I took it," she says. "Right now, I am trying methotrexate for the fifth time, and perhaps it will work. I have had a very good 2 months."

Samantha is not afraid of becoming addicted to painkillers. "I am very careful about what I take, and when. I hurt too much to experience any kind of high," she reflects.

Samantha's excellent relationship with her rheumatologists demonstrates that good medical care for a complex disease such as rheumatoid arthritis is based on a true partnership between doctor and patient. During the past 20 years, Samantha has had to deal with more than one arthritis specialist. When her all-time favorite physician relocated to the National Institute of Arthritis and Musculoskeletal and Skin Diseases in Bethesda, Maryland, she almost moved to Washington herself.

From the beginning, Samantha's arthritis has been atypical and unremitting. She experiences unusually severe inflammatory flares when a part of her body simply gives out and she cannot even stand up unaided. Once, when Charlie was still an infant, Samantha could not get to him when he woke up in the middle of the night. It was a terrible night for the two of them and Samantha swore that it would never happen again. After that, she made sure that crutches, a walker, and other self-help devices were within reach. Today, she parks her electric scooter next to her bed.

Samantha knows that her disease was hard on Charlie. "I worried about him growing up feeling responsible for me," she says. He now works full-time at a New York brokerage firm. He is 20 and has his own apartment. Samantha hopes that he realizes how important he is to her. "My son makes me smile," Samantha says. "Having to care for him made me get up in the morning."

Ten years ago, Samantha had breast cancer, and a few years ago, she went into kidney failure. "I wish that I could trade in my body," she says. Her body perhaps, but not her spirit. Like many other people with rheumatoid arthritis, her spirit is indomitable.

"It is so easy to become a patient," Samantha explains. "I refuse that role. I am me." Over the years, she has become softer: "The disease has humanized me. It has brought good people into my life, though I do get impatient when they complain about unimportant things in their lives. Nevertheless, I have learned to ask for help when I need it. I have learned to leave things undone. Nobody can help me when the pain is extreme, but I have learned to deal with it.

"When Charlie was small, my mother was distant. Today, when I am in pain, she is a real help. She is 85 years old now and lives in California. It's 3 hours earlier there, so I can call her in the middle of the night and complain. She had to learn to simply listen, not to mother me, not to promise that things will be better, and not feel sorry for me.

"Ten years ago, I started to sing. I discovered the healing power of hymns and black choral music, and I branched out from that. Friends come over and sing with me. I sing when I hurt and when I feel good. I wish that I could join a chorus, but my disease is too unpredictable for that. I also write poetry when I hurt. The first line always reflects my panic, but gradually as I write, the mood of the poem lifts.

"When I am in pain, time passes very slowly. I watch a clock and it barely moves. Distances, like a long hallway, look totally overwhelming when I hurt.

"I guess it is the unpredictability of the disease that is hardest to take. I don't even know what part of my body will be affected next. I find it hardest to deal with in between pain. When the pain is extreme, I know that I will have to wait it out, and when I feel good, I feel good.

"Sometimes I truly wish that I were rich enough not to work. Chronic disease is awfully expensive. I have a decent salary and good insurance. But still, there are taxis and drugs and deductibles and inlays for my shoes and phone bills...There is no end to it. But basically I know that my work is important to me. I go to the office when I feel good and work at home when I don't."

SERENA P.

You cannot tell from looking at her that 40-year-old Serena has severe, unremitting rheumatoid arthritis. She is perfectly groomed and greets everyone with a warm smile. She is scared of her disease because she watched her mother suffer from it.

Serena worked as a shoe sales clerk when her feet started giving out. She went to a podiatrist, who said that she had fallen arches. Soon, however, the pain spread to her ankles, knees, hips, and shoulders. She went to the emergency room at her local hospital. An increased sedimentation rate and a positive rheumatoid factor confirmed what Serena already suspected: She had rheumatoid arthritis.

Serena tried every drug developed for arthritis: ibuprofen, Voltaren, naproxen, prednisone, Plaquenil, ketoprofen, minocycline, methotrexate...Some of these drugs helped, some made her sick, and some scared her. "[Methotrexate] helped, but my hair was falling out and I was really getting scared," she recalled.

Serena's worst joint is her hip. "It keeps me from sleeping at night. I just can't seem to get comfortable." She will have hip surgery, but her muscles are weak from disuse. She needs to strengthen the muscles surrounding her hip as well as her arm muscles so that she can walk on crutches. Currently, she goes to physical therapy twice a week.

Serena is an expert at doing things for herself. Her toilet is equipped with a raised seat, and her shower has a stool. She puts on her stockings with garters attached to elastics and uses a long shoehorn for her shoes; she picks objects off the floor with a scissor-like reacher.

She, too, does not want to be a patient. "The hospital would send an ambulette for me," Serena explains, "but I prefer taking the subway." She keeps a spotless home for her brother and has as much fun as she can.

"I love to dance to all kinds of music—fast, rhythmic, slow. I can only dance 30 minutes or so, then I have to rest. I play cards almost every night.

"I have many friends and talk to them about my disease. I tell my fellow sufferers to stay strong, to keep their clinic appointments, and not to listen to quacks.

"Everybody always tells you that they know how to cure your arthritis. I do some of the stuff they recommend, like drinking herb teas or garlic, but I really know better.

"They tell me that I am much too young to have arthritis. I sometimes think so, too, but ever since I was a child, I figured that I would get arthritis. My mother came down with rheumatoid arthritis when she was 23 years old, and my grandma down in Alabama had some kind of arthritis. So I was not surprised when it hit me, too."

"I wish that I could go back to work," she told her physical therapist during her twice-weekly sessions. Then she lowered her expectations: "Perhaps it will at least be easier to keep house after they fix my hip," she sighed. Then she stretched out on the exercise mat and worked hard at strengthening her joints under the watchful eye of the therapist.

THE NEW APPROACH TO ARTHRITIS CARE

Though their arthritis varies in extent and intensity, the patients in this chapter share important characteristics:

◆ They are well informed about their disease.

◆ They trust their physicians.

◆ They are the captain of their medical team.

◆ They are in control, which is particularly important when dealing with an unpredictable, painful disease such as rheumatoid arthritis.

Control does not mean that you should go it alone. Effective management always rests on picking able partners. Before helping you to understand what is currently known about rheumatoid arthritis, let us provide you with the following 10 guidelines that will allow you to be a confident, empowered patient who will triumph over your disease:

1. Select your physician carefully.

2. Prepare for visits to the doctor's office.

3. Be well informed.

4. Obtain your medical reports.

5. Understand your drug therapy.

6. Understand your health insurance.

7. Maintain your treatment regimen.

8. Fight depression.

9. Keep an open mind.

10. Accept the fact that you are suffering from a chronic disease that requires some lifestyle modifications.

1. Select Your Physician Carefully

This is your most crucial decision, and it has unfortunately become more difficult with the advent of managed care.

It is absolutely essential that you like and trust your physician. Research has proven that patients suffering from rheumatoid arthritis always feel better after they have seen their physician, even if their treatment has not been altered.

Your physician should be associated with a good hospital. Most RA patients require physical therapy. Some may require occupational therapy, surgery, or other services from specialists. Your life will be simpler when these services are available at the hospital with which your physician is associated.

2. Prepare for Visits to the Doctor's Office

Visits to the doctor are stressful. You and your physician are busy people. To efficiently use your time, prepare a list of what you wish to discuss with your doctor (see Chapter 2).

3. Be Well Informed

You must become an informed consumer of medical care. Information about health and disease has exploded during the past decade. The bookstore shelves are bulging with good and bad self-help books. Television bombards arthritis patients with ads for over-the-counter medicines. Medical advice pours from the Internet. Newspapers, magazines, and specific disease-oriented newsletters keep you abreast of the latest developments. (For sources of information, Web sites, etc., see Appendix A) Be critical about this massive amount of information. If in doubt, discuss it with your physician.

Knowledge is important because your physician will insist that you participate in important decisions concerning your treatment. In addition, some aspects of medical care have become confrontational and sometimes even adversarial. Today, patients must sign informed consent forms before undergoing certain procedures such as surgery or taking certain experimental medications.

However, do not let these informed consent forms scare you unnecessarily. By law, every new drug consent form has to list every side effect it may cause; surgical consent forms must list every possible mishap. Taking the most cautious route may not always be the best option. To prevent permanent joint damage, rheumatologists often opt for aggressive treatment early in the course of the disease.

4. Obtain Your Medical Reports

It is helpful to obtain copies of your laboratory tests, X rays, and other information pertaining to your health. At first, the information may seem overwhelming, but it will start to make sense as you become an expert. After a while, you may recognize that your sedimentation rate, which is an indicator of inflammation (see Chapter 5), has dropped after taking a new type of medication. This clear indication of decreased disease activity may help you put up with some discomfort caused by a new treatment.

5. Understand Your Drug Therapy

Drug therapy for rheumatoid arthritis is both essential and complex. Moreover, and fortunately, entirely new drugs for the treatment of rheumatoid arthritis are in an advanced developmental stage, and your drug regimen may change. Drugs, however, are always double-edged swords. Chapter 6 provides information on how to take drugs safely.

6. Understand Your Health Insurance

It almost seems that red tape is overwhelming medical care. Doctors, nurses, and other medical personnel are spending valuable time figuring out patients' insurance coverage. You must know whether your policy covers drugs, physical therapy, massage, acupuncture, counseling, self-help devices, home health care, and so forth.

In the event that you must (or can) switch health insurance plans, opt for one that covers your particular needs.

7. Maintain Your Treatment Regimen

As an empowered patient it behooves you to stick to your treatment plan, which usually encompasses:

Drugs

Exercise

Rest

Weight maintenance (or control)

Good nutrition

Discuss any proposed changes with your physician. Inform your health care team of major noncompliance so that the omission can be factored into the evaluation of the treatment plan.

8. Fight Depression

Rheumatoid arthritis can be depressing. It is often accompanied by chronic pain. Its sufferers often have to abandon or limit favorite activities including sports, dancing, long walks, and even career options. Treatment is expensive and time-consuming, as are the lifestyle changes you may have to make.

Fortunately, many people suffering from rheumatoid arthritis are determined. Many of these people refuse to be victims, and none of those we have met in this chapter have been defeated by their disease.

9. Keep an Open Mind

Any patient suffering from rheumatoid arthritis owes a debt of gratitude to Sir John Charnley, M.D., who developed the artificial hip in a small hospital in Brighton, England, during the late 1950s. The first total hip replacement in the United States was performed in New York City during the late 1960s. Today, more than 300,000 hips and knees are replaced annually in the United States.

Initially, your doctors will do their utmost to prevent extensive joint damage. If the disease, nevertheless, manages to destroy one or more joints, you have the option of having it repaired. Total joint replacement surgery and repair of hips, knees, shoulders, elbows, finger joints, and so forth is like an insurance policy. Today, it is the exceptional patient with rheumatoid arthritis who will end up being totally disabled.

10. Accept Rheumatoid Arthritis in Your Life

Coping with RA is difficult. Most of us either become overly concerned or stubbornly fail to make allowances for pain and disability. Neither approach is helpful. Finding a balance between what you can do and what is too much is a difficult but most effective approach.

ONWARD AND UPWARD

You are now ready to tackle *The Hospital for Special Surgery Rheumatoid Arthritis Handbook*. The authors hope that it will help you navigate through old and new available treatments. You will not need all the information presented. As a matter of fact, it is likely that as medical knowledge about rheumatoid arthritis increases, treatment will become less complex. There is even some talk about finding an RA vaccine that will protect those at risk from developing overt disease. Until that red-letter day arrives, we hope that this book will become a trusted friend.

2

Your Doctor, Your Partner

This chapter reviews an initial overall treatment plan for RA. The tests, drugs, and other particulars mentioned in this chapter are detailed in subsequent chapters and defined in the glossary.

HENRY S.[1]

When he was 44 years old, Henry's shoulder started to hurt. He consulted an orthopedic surgeon, who diagnosed tendinitis (inflammation of a tendon). Henry received a few local injections of steroids, conscientiously applied cold packs to his shoulder, and took six ibuprofen pills a day.

Six months later, the pain in the shoulder was still there. In addition, both of Henry's legs hurt badly. Henry, who previously had gotten by reasonably well on 6 hours of sleep, was always tired. He was also losing weight.

Henry wondered if he might have gotten Lyme disease while vacationing at Martha's Vineyard. His doctor thought otherwise. He ordered a few more laboratory tests. Henry's *sedimentation* rate (a good measure of the level of inflammation) was high and he tested positive for rheumatoid factor. The orthopedic surgeon suggested that Henry consult Dr. R., a rheumatologist.

---

[1]Henry S. is a real patient. His name and certain details have been changed to protect his privacy.

Your Doctor, Your Partner ♦ 19

THE INITIAL CONSULTATION

A generation or two ago, the relationship between doctor and patient was more clear-cut. The doctor—most often a male—was clearly in charge and was totally responsible for the patient's well-being. Chances were that if a patient was diagnosed with severe arthritis, the doctor prescribed some drugs and told him or her to take it easy. Perhaps he recommended a spa. The patient trusted the doctor and swallowed whatever pills were prescribed. Neither the patient nor the doctor were concerned about their respective roles. Before the 1950s, the options for treating arthritis were quite limited.

Now matters are entirely different. Not only do doctors have choices, but they insist that their patients participate in decisions regarding their treatment. Many of the drugs routinely prescribed for RA are potent and can have serious side effects.

The approach to the treatment of RA has radically changed. In the past, the treatment regimen began with the lowest amount of the least potent drug available. Patients were started on aspirin and other nonsteroidal anti-inflammatory drugs (NSAIDS) such as ibuprofen. If they did not provide relief, the doctor would prescribe a more potent agent such as corticosteroids, gold injections, and other slow-acting agents (see Chapter 8).

Times have changed. By studying the records of thousands of patients, researchers have come to the conclusion that permanent joint damage occurs very early in the course of RA. Therefore, doctors now treat RA aggressively as soon as it is diagnosed. (This approach, which often minimizes the damage wrought by a particular disease, is also used in heart disease, cancer, AIDS, and many other disorders.)

The diagnosis of RA is still not as simple and as straightforward as it could be. There is no single blood test that provides a positive or negative diagnosis. Also, the most frequent major complaint, joint pain, can be caused by a host of other disorders. Nevertheless, by evaluating a combination of factors in an orderly manner, the physician can come up with an accurate diagnosis on which to base an initial treatment plan. This plan can be modified as additional information becomes available.

RA is a highly variable disease. Some patients arrive in the doctor's office with mild discomfort; others are dreadfully distressed and require immediate relief. The initial visit(s) usually proceeds as follows:

♦ Taking a detailed medical history

♦ Doing a complete physical examination

◆ Ordering diagnostic tests (imaging, laboratory tests)

◆ Initiating medical treatment

Physicians are very busy people and medical visits are stressful. It is usually helpful to review the procedure for the initial visit before arriving for the consultation (Table 2–1).

THE MEDICAL HISTORY

Symptoms

Onset of pain: When did you first notice the pain? Did it start suddenly or develop in the course of weeks or months?

TABLE 2-1. Preparation for the Initial Doctor's Visit

Symptoms	Describe your symptoms as accurately as you possibly can. Did they start suddenly? Slowly? When do you hurt most? At night? In the morning? After you exercise? How do you sleep at night? Are you tired during the day? Do you have morning stiffness, and, if so, how long does it last? Has your weight changed? Do you have fever?
Family history	Try to gather information about whether anyone else in your family has had arthritis. What kind? At what age? How severe? What therapy did they receive?
Medications	Make a list of all the drugs you presently take. Include those that you take only occasionally and those you buy without prescription. What are you presently taking for your joint problems, at what dosage, and for how long? Report any adverse and/or positive effects.
Exercise, rest	Describe your lifestyle. Describe activities you cannot do or do with difficulty (walking, running, raising arms, getting out of chairs, etc.). Compare your activities of daily living now with 6 months before your problem(s) began.
Questions	Ask about your diagnosis. (Since the physician may not yet have a definite answer, ask when you will find out.) When you receive a definite diagnosis, ask the doctors about your medical outlook. Discuss any fears and apprehensions you may have. Discuss treatments you believe may relieve your arthritis. Ask your physician for additional information about your disease and the various therapies used to treat it.

Type of pain: Is the pain intense? Dull? Localized? Do you hurt all over? How long does it last? When is it most severe? In the morning? During the day? At night? When you exercise? After you exercise? When you are resting?

Location of pain: Which joints hurt: neck, back, arms, wrists, fingers, hips, knees, feet? Which of these joints, if any, are swollen, red, or warm?

Pattern of pain: Does the pain occur in both knees, both hips, both pinkies, both wrists (etc.)?

Fatigue: Do you have trouble sleeping? Do you feel excessively tired? When? How many hours after you get up?

Mobility: Do you sometimes feel as if your body has "jelled"? When does this feeling occur? In the morning? After sitting for a while?

How far can you walk without getting tired or without hurting (think in terms of city blocks)? Can you climb stairs? Can you get up easily out of an armchair, out of an armless chair, from the floor, from a bed, from the toilet, out of the bathtub, and from a car? Can you bend down and pick up things from the floor? Can you turn faucets on and off?

Lifestyle: Much time will be spent on identifying the extent to which the disease interferes with your normal lifestyle. Does the disease keep you from doing things you normally do (activities of daily living, or ADL) such as combing your hair, shaving, cutting toenails, tying shoelaces, opening cans, accessing the toilet, closing buttons, getting groceries and books from high shelves, and so on?

Does your stiffness and/or pain interfere with your professional performance? Is your job at risk, and, if so, why? Has your present complaint impacted your usual physical activity (sports, exercise, walking, hiking, jogging, etc.)? Does your complaint interfere with your sex life? Are you depressed?

Other Medical Problems

Your physician must know about your other medical problems (past or present) including heart disease, hypertension, diabetes, infections, stomach trouble, previous hospitalizations and/or surgeries. Some of these diseases may impact on the proposed treatment. Because your current complaint may be indicative of other types of arthritis, a rheumatologist will be particularly concerned about:

◆ Skin rashes

◆ Fever

◆ "Sandy" feeling, itchy, dry, or red eyes

- Dry mouth
- Muscle weakness
- Changes in the color of your fingers upon exposure to cold

Medications

Effective treatment of RA rests on the availability of powerful medications. A physician can choose from about 50 different medicines. Since you may be taking drugs to manage other medical problems and different medications may interfere with one another, it is crucial that you provide the physician with the names of all the medications you are taking (prescription and over the counter), including

- Those taken occasionally (sleeping pills, allergy pills)
- Mood-altering drugs such as Prozac
- Birth-control pills
- Hormone replacements
- Stimulants and social drugs including alcohol
- Homeopathic remedies purchased at health food stores or elsewhere
- Vitamins
- Calcium and vitamin D
- Glucosamine and chondroitin sulfate

Be sure to report any drug allergies you may have. Chapter 6 provides basic information on medications.

Family History (Genetic Predisposition)

Rheumatic diseases such as RA run in the family. Try to remember whether anyone in your family had rheumatoid arthritis or any other rheumatic disease. Provide as many details as you can about who had the disease, when it was first diagnosed, its severity, and treatment, especially if it was successful.

THE PHYSICAL EXAMINATION

The physician will do a complete physical, including taking blood pressure and pulse rate, and listening to the heart and lungs. Much time will be spent on examining joints, feeling their warmth, observing how they function, and asking you how much they hurt while you bend, walk, and stretch. These measurements are a baseline and will be used to evaluate the effect of therapy.

The following factors are used to evaluate the degree to which RA affects your joints:

- *Joint function:* This criterion is subdivided into active and passive motion. To evaluate active motion, the physician will, for instance, have you flex (bend) a finger. To evaluate passive motion, the physician will bend the same finger. Some physicians may measure this movement with a goniometer (angle-measuring device).

- *Joint swelling:* RA causes a thickening of the synovial membrane that lines the joint capsule, as well as fluid accumulation (joint effusion). Both cause the joint to swell. A skilled physician is able to detect even minor swellings by pressing the joint with the fingers. Some of the larger joints (knees) may be measured with a tape.

- *Painful joints:* An inflamed joint will hurt when pressed.

The number of joints affected by RA is an indication of the activity of the disease and will be used as a guide to therapeutic response. Most typically, RA affects joints symmetrically (e.g., the same two joints of the right and left hand).

LABORATORY TESTS

The physician will order routine laboratory tests including hemoglobin levels, erythrocyte sedimentation rate (ESR), rheumatoid factor (RF), C-reactive protein (CRP), and others. Some of these measurements are indicative of inflammatory diseases. (For more details, see Chapter 5.) During ongoing treatment these tests will be used to evaluate RA activity and therapeutic response. Table 2–2 presents the guidelines of the American College of Rheumatology for the diagnosis of RA. While these criteria are used to standardize the diagnosis in RA studies, you may be interested in the information used by your doctor in making the diagnosis.

BACK TO HENRY S.

Let us now return to Henry S., the 44-year-old patient who we left on the doorstep of Dr. R., a rheumatologist.

TABLE 2-2. Medical Information Used in the Diagnosis of RA*

Morning stiffness	Morning stiffness lasting at least 1 hour.
Arthritis of 3 or more joints	At least 3 joints out of a possible 14 areas must appear swollen upon physical examination for at least 6 weeks.
Arthritis of the hand	Swelling of wrist or finger joints.
Symmetric arthritis	Simultaneous involvement of the same joint(s) on both sides of the body for at least 6 weeks.
Rheumatoid nodules	Subcutaneous (under the skin) bony lumps over or near the joints.
Rheumatoid factor	Positive.
Radiographic changes	Changes typical of RA as seen on X rays or by other imaging techniques.

*No single test or symptom is specific for RA. The American College of Rheumatology (ACR) considers the presence of four or more of these factors as a positive diagnosis for RA. Changes in these criteria are used to evaluate disease activity. For example, a decrease in the number of painful, inflamed joints and a decrease in CRP indicate less active disease and/or the effectiveness of a particular drug.

"When the orthopedic surgeon told me that he suspected that I suffered from RA, I realized that I had never heard of that disease," Henry S. recalled. "But when I told my parents about it, my father reminded me that my young nephew suffered from juvenile rheumatoid arthritis. My mom remembered that her cousin, Ada, had rheumatoid arthritis. So the disease definitely runs in my family."

Fortunately, Henry was not easily discouraged: "Until then I had been blessed with excellent health. Even now, I am not afraid, but I am tired and weary of having to deal with all that stuff.

"As soon as I knew that I suffered from RA, I educated myself. I read all I could, and that was extremely helpful."

After some additional diagnostic tests, Dr. R. initiated aggressive therapy. To begin, he prescribed 8 milligrams per day of methylprednisolone, a corticosteroid (see Chapter 9). These drugs do not change the course of RA, but they suppress pain and inflammation. Henry started to feel better.

Dr. R. also started Henry on a disease-modifying antirheumatic drug (DMARD; see Chapter 8). Of the many different drugs available, Dr. R. picked methotrexate. Before the 1980s, this drug was best known as a chemotherapeutic agent for cancer therapy. Though this sounds scary, it is crucial to realize that the dose (amount of drug) used for the treatment of RA is much lower than the dose used in cancer therapy. Unlike older DMARDs, methotrexate acts relatively rapidly, its beneficial effects becoming apparent within 3 to 6 weeks instead of 3 to 6 months for gold, another commonly used drug.

Dr. R. started Henry at 7.5 milligrams of methotrexate a week. Every month the doctor checked Henry carefully to determine whether the drug caused any ill effects and whether the activity of Henry's RA was abating.

Two laboratory tests provide important information about disease activity: the erythrocyte sedimentation rate (ESR) and the C-reactive protein (CRP). Both provide information on the level of inflammation (see Chapter 5). During the initial months of treatment, Henry's ESR remained high, and his CRP also remained elevated.

Dr. R. gradually increased Henry's dose of methotrexate from 7.5 mg/week, to 10 mg/week, to 12.5 mg/week, to 15 mg/week. Henry was instructed to take the total weekly dose in three installments at 12-hour intervals. "At first I did not understand this unusual way of taking my medication," Henry recalled, "and I made a mistake. Then Dr. R. explained that treating the RA with a large dose given within 36 hours once a week helps to strike the right balance between safety and controlling the inflammation."

The doctor also added 100 mg/day of cyclosporine. Treating RA with more than one DMARD is an option chosen by many rheumatologists.

After 3 months, Henry's disease finally responded. His ESR and his C-reactive protein decreased. His fatigue also decreased, though he never recovered the stamina he had before he became ill. Gradually, Henry's need for sleep decreased from 10 hours per night to 8 hours per night, and the duration of morning stiffness decreased from all morning to only 15 minutes. Dr. R. is weaning Henry off the steroids, and Henry continues to take 600 mg of ibuprofen instead of the 2400 mg he used to take. He makes sure to take the medication with food.

Henry is exercising cautiously. "Even when I was quite ill, I loved the warm, therapeutic pool at my health facility. My doctor suggests that I do more than that. This summer I shall start to work out under the supervision of a physical therapist."

The case of Henry S. is fairly typical, though other physicians might approach his disease somewhat differently. So much depends on the activity and severity of the RA at the time of diagnosis, the initial manifestations, the level of functional limitation, and the age of the patient. There is increasing evidence that early intervention with slow-acting DMARDs reduces ultimate joint destruction and improves patients' functional abilities. Even though such decisions are important, remember that joints do not deteriorate overnight and a treatment plan will be modified by your physician after evaluating your response to therapy.

YOU AND YOUR DOCTOR

Like Henry S., most patients suffering from RA will eventually be seen by a rheumatologist. A visit to a new doctor is important. It is the beginning of a partnership. You will have to decide whether you like and trust this physician, whether he or she listens to you, and whether your questions are answered completely in language that you understand. Also, does your physician consider medical costs and use your resources wisely?

Discovering that you suffer from a chronic, potentially disabling disease is traumatic. Remember that once the disease is under control, most patients lead normal, productive lives.

Given the complexity of medical care today, involving health maintenance organizations (HMOs) and other restrictions, it may be difficult for you to locate a physician you trust. Persevere in your efforts. By and large, rheumatologists are caring people, and you are likely to have a rewarding, lasting doctor–patient relationship. The rheumatologist will be only one member of the team that cares for you and your RA. The team also includes nurses, physical and occupational therapists, surgeons, and others. For details, see Chapter 3.

Information about diseases and drugs, successes and horror stories, abounds. Because arthritis encompasses a variety of disorders, most patients receive well-intentioned advice from friends and family. Most of these people will not know that RA is quite different from osteoarthritis, the most common and familiar form of the disease. It is especially important that you be well informed about your disease and learn to identify valuable information. If indicated, you can discuss suggested remedies with your health care providers. You can also contact the Arthritis Foundation for information. The Arthritis Foundation is a voluntary health agency that provides free information on its national hotline at 800–283–7800 and on the World Wide Web at www.arthritis.org. It has chapters throughout the United States. You can also get information from the American College of Rheumatology's (ACR) Web site: www. rheumatology.org and HSS's, rheumatologyhss.org.

Initiating Therapy

During the first visit, especially if your disease is very active and your joints are severely inflamed, your physician may consider initiating therapy with one of the powerful DMARDs. This approach is particularly indicated for patients incapacitated by moderate disease, as well as for those in whom the RA seems aggressive.

Treatment Plan

RA is a highly variable disease and treatment is individualized (see Table 2-3). When the disease is first diagnosed, it is difficult to completely predict its course and outcome, though certain symptoms may indicate whether the disease is likely to be mild or aggressive. Your physician will craft your therapy carefully, taking this and other important medical and social factors into consideration.

TABLE 2-3. Initial Treatment Plan

Diagnostic evaluation (This initial evaluation will serve as a baseline to evaluate the severity of the disease, your overall health, and the effectiveness of the basic treatment plan.)	• Medical history • Physical evaluation • Imaging of affected joints • Laboratory evaluation (rheumatoid factor, hemoglobin, C-reactive protein, erythrocyte sedimentation rate, general blood-screening tests)
Drug therapy	• Fast-acting • Nonsteroidal anti-inflammatory drugs (NSAIDs) • Disease-modifying antirheumatic drugs (DMARDs) • Immunosuppressants • Corticosteroids (to bring symptoms under control)

Medications

Three classes of medications play a major role in the management of RA.

◆ *Nonsteroidal anti-inflammatory drugs (NSAIDs):* These drugs, for example, aspirin and ibuprofen, suppress inflammation and control pain. The effect of these agents occurs more quickly than that of the DMARDs, with maximal action in 2 to 3 weeks. The use of these medications for pain and muscle aches is so common that you have probably taken an over-the-counter NSAID on your own, even before consulting a rheumatologist (see Chapter 7).

◆ *Disease-modifying anti-rheumatic drugs (DMARDs):* These drugs, for example, methotrexate, gold, etanercept, infliximab, azathioprine, cyclosporine, leflunomide, and D-penicillamine, are able to modify the course of RA, which is an action not shared with the NSAIDs. It will take weeks or months for these drugs to modify the activity of the disease—that is, to improve function, suppress inflammation, and decrease or stop joint damage. Depending on how you respond to a particular drug, your physician may try more than one until the desired goal is achieved (see Chapter 8).

◆ *Corticosteroids:* These powerful hormone-like drugs such as prednisone are used, often for a limited time period, to suppress inflammation (see Chapter 9).

Analgesics such as codeine, narcotics, antiulcer drugs such as Tagamet, and a host of other agents that minimize pain or counter the deleterious side effects of the primary medications may also be prescribed.

Surgery

Surgery is not necessary for most patients suffering from RA. Yet it is impossible to overestimate the blessing that effective surgery represents for those who need it as part of their overall rehabilitation program. Before total hip replacement surgery was performed in the United States, patients suffering from extensive hip disease were totally disabled. Today, hip and knee replacement surgery is almost routine. Other joints damaged by RA can also be repaired or replaced.

Your medical team will help you decide whether surgery is a good option. You, the captain of the team, will have to make the final decision. Factors to take into account before making such an important decision are considered in Chapter 16. Major surgical procedures used for patients suffering from RA are reviewed in Chapters 17, 18, and 19.

Rest and Joint Protection

Since fatigue is one of the major symptoms of RA, regularly scheduled rest periods should become part of your daily routine.

Inflamed joints are extremely vulnerable and should be protected as much as possible. Canes and walkers take pressure off hips and knees. A splint, worn at night, protects wrist and finger joints; a soft neck collar or a cervical pillow protects the cervical spine; a carefully adjusted chair reduces back strain; and labor-saving devices reduce stress on hand joints (see Chapter 12).

Exercise

Even though it is time-consuming, exercise plays a major part in the treatment of RA. Exercises preserve mobility, reduce pain, and strengthen the muscles surrounding the affected joints. In addition, exercises maintain cardiovascular health, improve overall physical fitness, reduce depression, and improve sleep (see Chapter 12).

Pain-Relief Techniques

Pain is the hallmark of RA. In addition to medications, it can often be mitigated through the local application of heat, cold, acupuncture, and other alternative forms of medicine (see Chapter 14).

Nutrition

Hippocrates, the father of medicine, was aware of the healing power of food. It took a long time for modern medicine to appreciate his wisdom. Chapter 11 reviews good nutrition and discusses the special needs of patients suffering from RA.

Companionship

A good support system plays an important part in the management of RA. In addition to your family and friends, you will profit from contact with other patients who battle the same disease. Your health team may put you in touch with others. The local chapter of the Arthritis Foundation may be able to refer you to a caring support group.

A GOOD LIFE IN SPITE OF RHEUMATOID ARTHRITIS

The biggest challenge for those with RA is to balance the demands of caring for joint problems with the need to lead a fulfilling, independent life. Chapter 14 offers examples of how other people suffering from RA have surmounted common difficulties.

3

What Is
Rheumatoid Arthritis?

━━━◈◈◈━━━

This chapter reviews basic facts about RA and provides information about other types of arthritis, health professionals who treat the disease, diagnosis, incidence, and progression.

Most people who discover that they suffer from rheumatoid arthritis are both puzzled and stunned. There is good reason for the confusion. There are many misconceptions about arthritis, for example:

◆ Arthritis, like the common cold, is not really a disease. How can it make you sick? Are you sure it's not in your head or it's not something else?

◆ Arthritis only affects the elderly!

◆ Arthritis can be cured by diet.

◆ If diet does not work, go see a chiropractor.

◆ If you still hurt, move to a warmer climate.

Let us review some facts and set the record straight.

A HUNDRED DIFFERENT DISEASES

Arthritis is a family name for a hundred different diseases. The common link between these disorders is painful joints. The cause for the joint involvement, however, varies from one disease to another.

In *osteoarthritis,* the most common form of arthritis, joint tissue wears down and degenerates. Another name for osteoarthritis is degenerative joint disease (DJD). In *gout,* sharp crystals resulting from a defect in the manner in which the body handles uric acid, a waste product, cause swelling and inflammation. In *infectious arthritis,* a microorganism inflames and may damage joint tissue. In *rheumatoid arthritis,* the joint is damaged by a chronic inflammation fueled by autoimmune processes.

Confusion also arises from the names used to describe RA and the other arthritides (plural of arthritis). The word *arthritis* comes from the Greek (*arthros* for "joint" and *itis* for "inflammation") and means "inflammation of the joints." For a very long time any disease associated with joint pain was simply called "arthritis."

Rheumatic is another term commonly used to describe these disorders. It comes from the Greek word *rheuma,* meaning "watery discharge," which might allude to the swollen, painful, "waterlogged" joints characteristic of the disease. More likely, however, is the fact that arthritis has always been linked with cold, wet weather.

Arthritis and *rheumatism* are not the only general terms used for this group of disorders. *Musculoskeletal diseases* refers to the fact that the arthritides involve the body's muscles and bones. *Connective tissue disease* indicates a systemic, inflammatory disorder such as RA or systemic lupus. The name comes from the characteristic inflammation of the tissues of the body that connect muscle, skin, bone, cartilage, blood vessels, tendons, ligaments, arteries, and the thin membranes enclosing the individual cells.

Collagen disease is a collective name for forms of arthritis in which the body attacks its own collagen-containing tissues, for example, systemic lupus erythematosus and dermatomyositis. Collagen is the most widely distributed protein constituent of connective tissue.

Two other names also help to define RA: *autoimmune* and *inflammatory.* For still unknown reasons, the immune system of RA patients malfunctions and targets the joints and other tissues, causing joint destruction and inflammation. Since ancient times, physicians were aware of the external signs of inflammation: redness, warmth, and swelling. Inside the body, an inflamed tissue is characterized by an accumulation of immune cells producing chemicals, which again contribute to cause joint damage. Putting these facts together makes RA both an autoimmune disorder and an inflammatory form of arthritis.

WHO GETS RHEUMATOID ARTHRITIS?

Another puzzling aspect of RA is that it is much more common in women than in men (3:1) and that the most common age of onset is between the ages of 30 and 50. Over the age of 60, the disease occurs with equal incidence in men and in women.

RA affects approximately 1 percent of the population over age 15. Indeed, the Arthritis Foundation estimates that in the United States a total of 2.5 million people suffer from this most common form of inflammatory arthritis. Each year, approximately 67 new cases of RA are diagnosed per 100,000 people in the United States. The prevalence of the disease increases with age.

RA occurs in the same frequency throughout the world, thereby demonstrating that neither climate nor diet alone plays a role in its genesis. Certain ethnic groups, however, are at greater risk than others. In some Native American groups, 5 to 6 percent of the population suffers from RA, suggesting that genetic predisposition plays a major role. The disease may also cluster in certain families. Alternatively, African Americans seem to be at somewhat lower risk than white Americans.

The rate at which RA affects the children of parents with RA is only 2 percent. Even in identical twins, the rate at which both have RA is 12 percent. Thus, genetics can only account for a part of the predisposition to RA. Some researchers suspect that an infection by a common virus or other environmental factors contribute to RA causation. Sixty-five percent of patients suffering from RA have a genetic marker called HLA-DR4. Because the remainder of those positive for the HLA-DR4 marker never develop RA, the appearance of active disease requires some other trigger factor.

In the future, a vaccine may protect persons positive for HLA-DR4 from developing active disease. Or, RA may turn out to be a group of slightly different diseases, each responding to different forms of therapy.

WHO TREATS RHEUMATOID ARTHRITIS?

Doctors specializing in the treatment of patients suffering from arthritis are called rheumatologists. Ideally, your principal physician will be a board-certified rheumatologist with good clinical judgment, knowledge of all currently available treatments, infinite patience, and a willingness to try new approaches if your current treatment is unsatisfactory.

The professional organization to which these specialists belong is the American College of Rheumatology (ACR), which will be mentioned frequently in this book. If you are in need of a rheumatologist, you may call ACR for a referral.

The voluntary health organization that concerns itself with all forms of arthritis is the Arthritis Foundation, which will also be mentioned frequently. The Arthritis Foundation has chapters throughout the United States and can provide you with names of rheumatologists.

Rheumatologists are in short supply. Your internist or family practitioner, however, is qualified to handle most aspects of your care and may refer you to a rheumatologist for a consultation or second opinion if necessary.

Treatment for this complex disease is usually delivered by a team of health professionals.

Nurses mastermind your care in and out of the hospital. Depending on the setting, nurses supervise your medication regimen, evaluate the results of your laboratory tests, and answer questions you may have about your treatment.

Physical therapists observe how you use your body, teach you how to exercise so as to preserve the function of the large joints affected by RA, help you develop an overall exercise plan, and, if necessary, provide you with canes and walkers.

Occupational therapists teach you to use your body in the most mechanically efficient manner possible, and to protect and exercise the small joints (i.e., hands and arms); make splints to protect your joints whenever necessary but especially during active flares; and help you solve problems with difficult tasks, for example, by providing you with self-help gadgets.

Orthopedic surgeons counsel you about surgical options. They repair and replace joints in which function has been limited by joint damage and/or because pain is intolerable.

Social workers may help you sort out emotional and financial problems associated with having a chronic disease, as well as problems with your health insurance or health maintenance organization (HMO). They can locate suitable rehabilitation facilities, home health care, transportation, and other essentials.

Dietitians develop personalized eating plans to help you put on or take off weight.

The most important member of your team, however, is *you,* the patient. The more determined you are that RA won't get you down, the better off you will be.

COST

RA is an expensive disease in terms of direct medical costs and indirect lost-time costs. According to government statistics, each year the disease accounts for 9 million physician visits and 250,000 hospitalizations. Its annual cost exceeds $8.7 billion. These figures are expected to increase. Many new and effective medications, such as tumor necrosis factor antagonists (see Chapter 8), are extremely costly.

Suffering from RA is time-consuming. Often, you will become discouraged and impatient with the time spent sitting in doctors' offices, filling out insurance forms, catering to your body, and doing your exercises. You'll hate losing time from work (RA accounts for $6.5 billion in lost wages annually) and taking medications that are sometimes ineffective. Even if you are lucky enough to have good insurance coverage, you'll spend extra money on cabs and other necessities.

Tell yourself that you have no choice. Think of all the wonderful people who suffered from RA. Did you know that Auguste Renoir, the most luminous of the Impressionists, suffered from RA during the last decades of his life?

DIAGNOSING RHEUMATOID ARTHRITIS

In the past, it commonly took months, even years, to obtain a definite diagnosis of RA. This was because the disease presentation is highly variable and sometimes its main symptoms are vague and nonspecific. Today, with improved physician education and greater access to information for the patient with joint pains, the diagnosis is made earlier and more quickly, and therapy is started sooner. Once the doctor suspects that a patient is suffering from RA, a diagnosis is usually forthcoming within a matter of weeks. Chapter 2 discusses criteria for RA diagnosis.

WHAT TO EXPECT

The course of RA is highly variable. Whereas some patients suffer from very aggressive disease, in others the disease is relatively mild. Currently it is estimated that 30 percent of patients have mild disease, varying from a return to apparent good health after a period of active disease to occasional flares separated by remissions.

The other 70 percent will develop chronic RA. Of these, 15 percent will suffer from aggressive, potentially crippling RA. These patients will tend to have a higher incidence of systemic (affecting the entire body) involvement and joint damage.

Mild disease is defined as a few inflamed joints, mild fatigue, and minimal limitation of function. Many actively inflamed joints, significant fatigue, and the early development of joint damage and functional limitation characterize severe RA. Because it is important to treat RA early and adequately, the aggressiveness of the treatment is proportional to the level of joint inflammation and limitation in function.

When instituted early, modern aggressive treatment clearly reduces joint damage and lessens the overall impact of the disease. Remember that joint damage does not occur overnight. Help is available. Chances are good that your disease can be controlled.

MONITORING THE DISEASE

Doctors need to monitor and assess their patients' status. Routine evaluations will indicate whether the disease is under control and whether the response to a new drug is good, bad, or indifferent. Table 3-1 lists common RA measurement tools.

Table 3-1. Routine Assessment Tools to Measure the Activity and Extent of RA

Use of the measurement tools: The medications and other components of your treatment regimen will be guided by your physician's assessment of the state of inflammation and functional limitation, ranging from mild to moderate to severe. He or she will ask you questions, examine you, and order laboratory tests and possibly X rays to categorize the state of your RA both at the beginning and throughout its course. Your therapy may change significantly over time based upon changes in the activity of your RA and its response to a treatment regimen. Eventually, your physician will develop a disease activity equation using the following pieces of information:

1. *Historical facts* (your answers to the physician's questions): This information will be taken into account by your physician:

    a. Duration of morning stiffness, in minutes or hours

    b. Level of joint pain, which can be measured on a scale, with **10 being the worst you can be** or how you were before starting the medication to **0 being no pain at all**

    c. Level of joint swelling using the same scale

    d. Level of fatigue using the same scale

    e. Overall level of function using the same scale

    f. Overall level of disease activity using the same scale

2. *Physical examination findings:* At each visit, your physician will examine all your joints to assess the amount of inflammation and function.

    a. Joint range of motion determined in degrees of range of motion

    b. Grip strength measured using a blood pressure cuff or by the finger squeeze test

    c. Number of swollen joints by assessing 28 to 68 joints

    d. Number of tender joints

3. *Laboratory and X-ray testing:* Laboratory and X-ray evaluations are not routinely performed at each visit, unless they are needed for monitoring of medications. However, often the rheumatologist will obtain baseline blood tests and possibly X rays in order to compare these results with later ones. A *complete blood count* assesses the following:

    a. *Hemoglobin level:* This is a determination of the oxygen-carrying protein in red blood cells. The hemoglobin level may decrease in the presence of active RA and is a good guide to the level of inflammation. Normal hemoglobin is 13–17 g% in men and 11.5–16.0 g% in women. The hematocrit is an alternative method, with normal levels being 35 to 44 percent.

(continued)

TABLE 3-1. *(continued)*

b. *Platelet count:* Platelets are cells that participate in blood coagulation (blood clotting). The level of these cells may increase in the presence of inflammation. Normal platelet counts range from 160,000 to 400,000.

c. *Erythrocyte sedimentation rate (ESR):* This test measures the rate at which red blood cells fall in a tube. In the presence of inflammation, proteins are increased in the blood. Thus, the red blood cells fall more quickly. Normal ESR is 20 millimeters per hour or less. ESR is a general guide to the level of inflammation, with higher levels representing more active disease.

d. *C-reactive protein (CRP):* Inflammation increases the level of CRP in the blood. This test is a bit more sensitive to changes in disease activity than ESR. However, ESR is a simpler and cheaper test, and thus it is used more frequently.

e. *Blood chemistry testing:* A screening blood test called SMA-12 allows the physician to assess the function of the kidney and liver as well as blood sugar and uric acid levels. These results can guide the doctor in choosing specific medications. These measurements also serve as a baseline for future comparison.

f. *Rheumatoid factor (RF):* The serum of 80 percent of RA patients contains antibodies called rheumatoid factors that react with other proteins called immunoglobulins (see Chapter 5). These autoantibodies are part of the autoimmune process and probably play some role in joint inflammation (antibodies are made against outside invaders; autoantibodies are made against a person's own tissues). Since RA is diagnosed primarily on clinical grounds, the absence of RF does not rule out the diagnosis. The test is a confirmation of the diagnosis.

g. *X rays:* The finding of joint erosion on an X ray, particularly early in the course of the disease, is a sign to the physician to be more aggressive with therapy. Thus, a baseline X ray of one hand or foot may be performed and then compared with other X rays done on a 6- to 12-month basis. The primary aim with all RA treatment is to modify disease, which means stopping the development of new erosions or having old ones heal.

4. *Health assessment questionnaire:* Questionnaires are available that measure the degree of disability and assess the psychosocial and functional level of patients. Some physicians have their patients fill out a questionnaire each time they are seen. The answers may alert the physician to a particular problem.

◆ CHAPTER ◆

4

How Rheumatoid Arthritis Affects the Body

———➤◉◄———

This chapter reviews the structure of the musculoskeletal system and describes how it is affected by rheumatoid arthritis.

The human body consists of about 300 individual bones, connected by more than 140 joints. To function, a joint also requires ligaments, tendons, and muscle tissue. Since some of these structures are the primary targets of RA, let us examine them in some detail.

BONES

Bones, the main structural support for the body, are composed of a mineral called hydroxyapatite and protein in the form of collagen. The mineral makes up 67 percent of bone and provides rigidity; the protein provides elasticity. As attested by the skeletons of dinosaurs, bones are built to last for millions of years. Dinosaurs, as well as Egyptian mummies, show evidence of osteoarthritis.

It was believed that bones were relatively inert once they were formed. Today, we know that bone is constantly turned over. This makes sense, since the body is able to repair a broken bone. Two special types of cells carry out remodeling and repair work: (1) The *osteoclasts* remove bone. (2) The *osteoblasts* form new bone.

Both types of cells participate in mending broken bones. Diseases that affect bone metabolism, including arthritis and osteoporosis, impact on the balance between osteoclasts and osteoblasts. Some of the medications used in the treatment of RA may affect the normal equilibrium between bone formation and bone loss.

Corticosteroids, for example, primarily stimulate the bone-removing osteoclasts, thereby promoting bone loss and osteoporosis. Many of these side effects can be managed successfully. Figure 4–1 shows the structure of a long bone. Note that toward the end a layer of subchondral bone and cartilage, both of which can be damaged by RA, cap the bone.

JOINTS

A joint is the place where two or more bones meet. Given the number of different tasks the skeleton must perform, it is surprising that nature evolved only three types of joints:

1. Synarthroidal or fibrous joints
2. Amphiarthroidal or cartilaginous joints
3. Diarthrodial or synovial joints

In synarthrodial joints, for example, those that separate the plates that form the skull, bones stay put with respect to one another. Synarthrodial joints are not affected by RA.

In amphiarthrodial joints, such as the intervertebral discs of the spinal column, the fibrocartilaginous material that separates the bones permits limited movement. Even though these joints wear, degenerate, and herniate, amphiarthrodial joints are not affected by RA.

The highly mobile diarthrodial or synovial joints are the target of RA.

Overall Joint Function

Joints provide both mobility and stability. Even without overt arthritis, the body becomes stiffer as it ages. The joints of a newborn are much more mobile than those of a 5-year-old. Exaggerated stiffness is the hallmark of any form of arthritis, and throughout this book there will be much emphasis on exercises that maintain mobility.

FIGURE 4-1. Schematic View of a Long Bone. Most bones of the skeleton are hollow cylinders constructed as follows:

The *shaft*. This central portion of the bone is very rigid. It consists of relatively unbending, dense connective tissue.

The *epiphysis*. Growth during the first 15 years of life takes place in the epiphysis, the ends of the bone.

Subchondral bone. Subchondral bone is found directly under the cartilage. It is more porous and is replaced more frequently by new bone than the more highly calcified bone of the shaft. Upon impact, subchondral bone can absorb some of the stress.

Articular cartilage. The collagen and proteoglycan fibrils within the cartilage are arranged to help evenly distribute the stress created by movement.

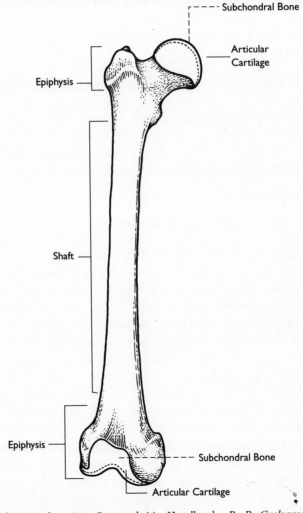

Overall Joint Architecture

The joints have a well-defined architecture. There is adequate space between the ends of the bones, permitting free, unimpeded movement. This perfect structure is destroyed during active disease. When the inflammation is active (see Chapter 5), white blood cells and inflammatory mediators (body chemicals that cause inflammation) migrate into the joint cavity, increasing the volume of the synovial fluid. The joint becomes painful and swollen, and the clear synovial fluid becomes cloudy. The thin synovial lining becomes swollen. The joint space may decrease due to prolonged exposure of its components to inflammation. Eventually the bony structure of the joint may become altered and the entire joint may become nonfunctional. Medications may slow or halt these degenerative processes.

What Joints Are Affected by Rheumatoid Arthritis

RA does not affect every synovial joint. The disease most often affects the small joints of the hands and feet, the hips, knees, elbows, and shoulders. Nobody knows why it spares some joints and affects others. As the disease progresses, more joints may become involved.

The Shape of Synovial Joints

The individual joints of the body are admirably adapted to their function. Ball-and-socket joints rotate, hinge joints open and close, and the carpal bones of the foot roll. Figure 4–2 illustrates some of the more commonly encountered synovial joints.

Some joints that move in one plane, such as the elbows and fingers, are true hinges. The rotating hip is a ball-and-socket joint, as is the shoulder. The wrist consists of several bones that act like a ball bearing, permitting a rolling type of motion. The thumb swivels. Previous generations of RA patients became crutch-, wheelchair-, or bed-bound once the disease had destroyed the function of a crucial joint. Today, joint damage can be prevented. However, in those patients who do develop limiting or painful joint disease, many joints can be replaced surgically. More information on specific joints will be reviewed in the chapters dealing with surgery.

FIGURE 4-2. Examples of Commonly Encountered Synovial Joints. *From* The Columbia Presbyterian Osteoarthritis Handbook, *R. P. Grelsamer and S. Loebl, eds. Macmillan, 1996. Reproduced with permission.*

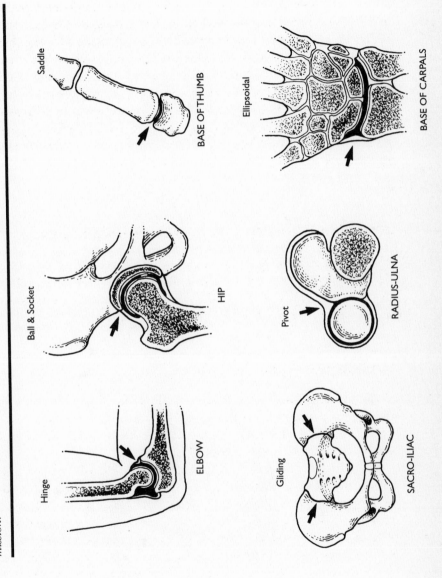

43

Overall Structure of a Synovial Joint and Its Capsule

Even though synovial joints come in various shapes, they basically have the same overall structure (see Fig. 4–3). To begin with, the entire joint is enclosed in a joint capsule consisting of *tough fibrous tissue* that keeps the bones in place and prevents the joint from overextending.

The fibrous capsule is lined by the thin *synovium*. In healthy individuals the synovium is extremely thin, often consisting of sheets of single cells, called *synoviocytes*. These cells produce clear, viscous synovial fluid. Essential nutrients are delivered to the synovium by microscopic blood and lymphatic vessels.

The ends of the bones that form the joint are covered by shock-absorbing *articular cartilage*. Anyone familiar with the gristle that connects a chicken drumstick with its thighbone knows what articular cartilage looks like. It is elastic, absorbing the impact of the body during

FIGURE 4-3. Schematic View of a Synovial Joint. A joint connects two or more bones. Note the articular cartilage that covers the ends of the bone. In a healthy joint the bones are separated by a well-defined joint space. The entire joint is enclosed by both a synovial membrane and a fibrous capsule. The synovial membrane secretes a viscous, clear fluid—the synovial fluid—which fills the joint cavity. *From* The Columbia Presbyterian Osteoarthritis Handbook, *R. P. Grelsamer and S. Loebl, eds. Macmillan, 1996. Reproduced with permission.*

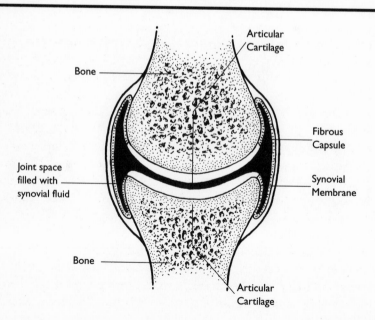

walking and other exercise, and it is extremely smooth. When healthy, articular cartilage is more slippery than ice, permitting joint surfaces to glide over one another effortlessly during an entire lifetime.

The tissues making up the articular cartilage are intricately organized. Cartilage consists of collagen and proteoglycans (20 to 35 percent of total weight) and fluid (65 to 80 percent). This water is responsible for the cartilage's elasticity. Cartilage acts like a sponge, absorbing water during relaxation, extruding it during impact. During almost any movement, this process is repeated over and over again, for instance, 50 or more times per minute during walking.

Like bone, articular cartilage is constantly turned over. Specialized cells, called *chondrocytes,* are dispersed throughout the cartilage, manufacturing collagen and proteoglycan. The chondrocytes are responsible for the formation, maintenance, and degradation of the cartilage.

In normal joints, a thin layer of *synovial fluid* covers the surface of the synovium and cartilage. The synovial fluid has the consistency of egg white and is rich in nutrients, oxygen, and hyaluronic acid. In certain forms of arthritis, including RA and infectious arthritis, the joint fluid is altered. During a diagnostic workup, the physician may remove a small amount of synovial fluid with a syringe and send it to the laboratory for analysis.

MUSCLES, TENDONS, LIGAMENTS, AND BURSAE

On its own the joint does not move. Muscles, tendons, and ligaments, collectively referred to as *soft tissues,* implement motion. Movement occurs via the contraction (shortening) of a muscle and the pulling of an attached tendon that moves over a joint. Both the ligaments, which attach bone to bone, and the tendons, which attach bone to muscle, consist of extremely fibrous cord-like tissues that can withstand much stress. Familiar tendons are the Achilles tendon of the foot and the outer elbow tendon, which causes "tennis elbow" when inflamed. Familiar ligaments are the cruciate ligaments of the knee. Ligaments and tendons contribute to joint mobility and stability, especially in exposed joints such as the knee.

Because these tissues are under extreme stress, they are cushioned by small synovial fluid-filled pouches called bursae. Both tendons and bursae can become inflamed, resulting in tendinitis and bursitis (note the ending *itis,* as in arthritis, which denotes inflammation).

The muscle mass surrounding any particular joint is closely related to the function of that joint. The mobile weight-bearing hip is embedded in, and protected by, a bulky mass of muscles, whereas the more peripheral joints, such as those found in the fingers, are much more vulnerable and exposed.

RA can lead to inflammation and even damage to tendons. Hand tendons can rupture as the disease progresses. Pain, however, may force patients to stop using an affected joint. Such disuse may rapidly lead to muscle atrophy (deterioration), which in turn aggravates the disease. Loss of muscle tissue may alter the proper joint alignment, resulting in disuse and eventually deformity. Thus, exercise plays a crucial role in the management of RA.

There is still another reason to maintain good muscle tone. Muscles absorb part of the stress that ordinary use places on a joint. This extra stress is easy to demonstrate. All of us are familiar with the painful impact that occurs when we stumble down an unanticipated curbstone.

SYMPTOMS OF RHEUMATOID ARTHRITIS OUTSIDE THE JOINTS

RA can affect the entire body. The most common general symptoms are fatigue, malaise, and weight loss. Even though the symptoms should lessen with successful treatment, they may never disappear completely.

Malaise and Fatigue

Malaise and fatigue are French words, the first meaning "not feeling up to par," the second meaning "being tired." Patients with RA are familiar with both. When RA is active, you may feel as if you have a chronic flu. Malaise and fatigue wax and wane with RA. Much effort will be spent in this book suggesting ways to deal with these manifestations.

Weight Loss

Weight loss is a common early manifestation of RA. It is caused by the systemic effect of the cytokines (tumor necrosis factor, TNF) and the interleukins (IL-6 and IL-1), which is discussed in Chapter 5. Body weight usually returns to normal when symptoms are controlled.

Other Organ Systems

In less than 10 percent of patients, RA can involve other internal structures or organs. Such manifestations are commonly referred to as extra-articular features of RA. These include the following abnormalities.

Blood

RA is often accompanied by anemia (a decreased number of red blood cells). This is most often caused by suppression of bone marrow resulting from the inflammatory process. The condition commonly improves as the disease is controlled. Anemia may also result from imperceptible blood loss caused by nonsteroidal anti-inflammatory drugs (NSAIDs) that irritate the gastrointestinal tract, promoting ulcers. (The problem can be identified by stool hemoccult testing.)

Eyes

Occasionally, patients may suffer from *sicca syndrome* characterized by dry eyes and/or dry mouth. Inflammation affects the glands that produce tears and/or saliva. Both symptoms are more annoying than dangerous. Symptoms can be aggravated by medications that contain antihistamines (cold medication, over-the-counter sleeping pills, allergy medication, and others).

Dry eyes are relieved by over-the-counter eye lubricants and/or artificial tears. A dry mouth requires excellent mouth hygiene. Though the sucking of candy relieves dry mouth, beware of sugar-laden sweets, which promote tooth decay.

Rheumatoid Nodules

About 20 percent of patients with RA develop small lumps under the skin around the elbow called *rheumatoid nodules.* These nodules are generally harmless, but if they interfere with normal function of the body, surgical removal is indicated. Rheumatoid nodules most often occur in patients with a potentially severe course of RA. Their presence may thus be an additional indication for aggressive therapy. In some patients, such nodules can be caused by methotrexate.

Chest and Lungs

Inflammation of the pleura (the membrane lining the chest) can occur, manifested by pain in the chest on deep breathing (pleurisy). The condition, most common in men with severe RA, responds to anti-inflammatory drugs. Lung involvement can rarely be due to RA itself or is sometimes a side effect of methotrexate therapy.

Heart

Very rarely the pericardium (the membrane enclosing the heart) may become inflamed in patients suffering from advanced RA. The condition usually responds to drug therapy.

Nerves

Joint and tendon swelling or damage may occasionally compress the nerves that transmit messages to various parts of the body. The best-known complication is carpal tunnel syndrome, which results from the compression of the median nerve that runs through the wrist. This can result in tingling and numbness in the affected part. The condition responds to splinting and occasionally to surgery.

Felty's Syndrome

This disorder is a rare complication characterized by a swollen spleen, low white blood cell count, recurrent infections, and leg ulcers. It tends to occur in patients with severe RA. Felty's syndrome often responds to disease-modifying antirheumatic drugs (DMARDs) such as methotrexate, leflunomide, and the anti-TNF medications (see Chapter 8). The administration of growth factors may also be helpful. If none of these measures work, and if the symptoms are severe, the physician may consider a splenectomy, which is successful in 50 percent of cases.

Rheumatoid Vasculitis

This inflammation of the blood vessels rarely occurs in patients suffering from RA. It can be minor or major depending on the blood vessels affected. A malignant life-threatening form occurs rarely and requires aggressive treatment with high doses of corticosteroids and strong disease-modifying antirheumatic drugs (DMARDs).

5

RA Immunity and Inflammation

—————◦《◎》◦—————

This chapter explores the immune system and explains how its malfunction can cause rheumatoid arthritis. The current concepts of immunity and immune mechanisms have been greatly simplified.

When we reviewed the multiple names for rheumatoid arthritis, we came across the terms *autoimmune disorder* and *inflammatory arthritis*. Put together, these two names actually describe the major characteristics of RA quite well. Both immunity and inflammation are part of the body's natural defense system, both malfunction in RA, and both are the targets of the drugs used to keep RA in check.

IMMUNITY

The importance of the immune system was highlighted in 1980 when physicians noted patients with an extremely rare form of cancer and an equally rare form of pneumonia. Within a matter of months, it was discovered that these disorders occurred in people whose immune system had been destroyed by a virus. The human immunodeficiency virus (HIV) that causes acquired immune deficiency syndrome (AIDS) had arrived.

AIDS underlined that an adequately functioning immune system is essential for survival. Not only does the immune system permit the body to fight off or recover from infection by various microorganisms, but it safeguards the body from developing a variety of diseases including cancer.

In RA, as well as in a number of other diseases, including type I diabetes, systemic lupus erythematosus (SLE), and ulcerative colitis, the immune system malfunctions and directs its fury against its own tissues. Some of the drugs (corticosteroids, methotrexate, cyclosporine) used to control RA work because they suppress the immune system. At present, these therapies are like swatting a mosquito with a sledgehammer. It is reasonable to believe that an increased understanding of the immune system will lead to more specific treatments. Indeed, a new class of biologic drugs such as Enbrel (etanercept), and Remicade (infliximab) which is a tumor necrosis factor antagonists, or monoclonal antibodies are now available or used experimentally.

The Dawn of Immunity

Long before the concept of immunity existed, physicians realized that most infectious diseases occur only once. This fact was almost obvious. Take smallpox, for example. In England, about the time of the American Revolution, smallpox was extremely common. One person out of every four contracting smallpox died, but those who survived never again came down with the disease.

At the time, Edward Jenner, a country physician, decided to explore a rumor claiming that people who had contracted cowpox, a rather mild disease, were protected from deadly smallpox. Jenner infected a few people with cowpox and demonstrated that they were indeed immune to smallpox. The word *vaccine* (from *vacca*, Latin for "cow") is a reminder of the many debts humanity owes the cow.

The smallpox vaccine was the world's first. Dozens more are available today, and many of the scourges of the past (yellow fever, polio, mumps, measles) are rare in advanced countries. Because of Jenner's vaccine, smallpox has been eliminated. Today, vaccines are being developed against a variety of noninfectious diseases, and it is hoped that someday we will have a vaccine against RA.

The scientific basis of immunity was developed about a century ago. By then, it was known that specific microbes cause disease and that during recovery from such an infection the body manufactures some protective substances. The causative agent was called *antigen* because it was able to *gene*rate the formation of an *anti*body. Many of the other terms used in immunology today, such as *complement, agglutination,* and *phagocytosis,* were coined by these early immunologists. The immune system turned out to be infinitely more complex than these early pioneers could have imagined.

The Organization of the Body

Living creatures consist of billions of individual cells. Some of these are knitted together in tissues such as the liver or the synovial lining of the joint capsule. Others, such as red and white blood cells, float around freely in body fluids (blood, synovial fluid, lymph, seminal fluid, etc.). Each type of cell carries out a specific job. Some—for example, the cells of the skeleton—provide structure. Muscle cells provide motion and nerve cells transmit messages. Many cells manufacture body chemicals such as hormones, enzymes, and antibodies. Coming back to the subject at hand, the job of the cells of the immune system is to protect the body from intruders such as viruses and bacteria.

Seventy percent of the entire body is fluid (water). Some of this fluid—for example, saliva, lymph, and plasma—surrounds the cells. In addition, each cell is a speck of fluid enclosed in a thin membrane that carefully monitors traffic between the outside of the cell and its interior. The fluid outside the cells is called the *extracellular fluid* and the fluid enclosed in the cell membrane is called the *intracellular fluid.*

The immune system is subdivided into the *humoral branch,* which identifies and attacks foreign substances in the extracellular fluid, and the *cellular branch,* which identifies and attacks foreign substances that have managed to penetrate the inside of the cell. Humoral immunity comes into play before cellular immunity. This makes sense when one likens a cell to a house. It stands to reason that it is less costly to catch a burglar outside the house (cell) than inside it, especially since the weapons used by cellular immunity usually end up destroying the entire "house."

The Organization of the Immune System

It may be helpful to compare the immune system to an army whose job is to protect the body from foreign invaders and safeguard the integrity of the body. Like most armies, the immune system has an array of foot soldiers, provides identification for the "legal residents" (self), has a highly developed communication system, and has a storehouse of specialized weapons. Let us look at these divisions in some detail.

The Foot Soldiers

The most important component of the immune system are the foot soldiers that confront the antigens. The foot soldiers consist of six types of leukocytes (white blood cells) that descend from identical stem cells produced by the bone marrow (see Fig. 5-1).

Four of these white blood cells (neutrophils, monocytes/macrophages, basophils, and eosinophils) are the shock troops that participate in the initial nonspecific immune defense; two white blood cells, the B and T lymphocytes, participate in the later defense. The shock troops produce mediators of inflammation, and the macrophages clean up cellular debris and attempt to engulf anything foreign. The cells of the immune system constantly patrol the body, identifying anything that does not seem to belong. They exchange information with each other, via chemical or cell-to-cell interaction, and, if indicated, develop a plan of action. Many of these white blood cells are short-lived and are constantly replaced. Most leukocytes die without having seen any action.

Identification of Self

In any skirmish, it is essential to distinguish between friend and foe, or to be more scientific between self and nonself. The self-cells of each individual are identified by permanent tags provided by proteins called major histocompatibility complex (MHC) markers.

There are two sets of MHC markers: Class I (MHC I) and Class II (MHC II). Each person has 6 out of at least 200 possible variants of MHC I and 8 of a possible 230 MHC II variants.

You do not have to be a mathematical genius to realize that humans come in an almost infinite number of MHC combinations. The only people who have the same markers are identical twins. These markers play a key role in organ transplantation medicine where physicians talk of "good matches" and "poor matches" depending on how many markers an organ donor and an organ recipient share.

When patrolling the body, the foot soldiers of the immune system ignore any cell earmarked with the person's own MHC marker (self-cells). Self-cells that are infected by a virus, however, are mercilessly destroyed.

Communication

As always, communication is subdivided into sending messages and receiving messages. To accomplish these tasks, the immune system utilizes *chemical messengers,* collectively referred to as soluble mediators (enablers) of immunity or immune modulators, which transmit information between cells; and *cell receptors,* which are able to interpret this information.

Most of the *soluble mediators of immunity* produced by the cells of the immune system are proteins. Some of these specialize in communication between cells; others participate in the elimination of the foreign invader; still others are involved in cleaning up cellular debris. Some cells of the immune system produce only one mediator whereas others secrete dozens. For example, during an immune response a macrophage produces a hundred different mediators, whereas each B lymphocyte produces only one very specific one. Relevant mediators are discussed in more detail in the section dealing with the immune response and in Table 5–1.

It is of interest that the body often produces two messengers with opposite effects. Take the prostaglandins, for example. Prostaglandin E2 promotes inflammation, whereas prostaglandin F reduces inflammation. Another well-known example is sugar metabolism. The hormone insulin promotes the storage of glucose, whereas glucagon promotes the release of glucose. A biological system controlled by two opposing messengers permits a healthy body to maintain itself in equilibrium. In disease, this finely tuned balance is often lost.

Receptors embedded in the membranes that enclose the cells receive and interpret messages from the outside. We have already encountered the tags of the histocompatibility complex. The receptors on the cell surface, however, also transmit information about the state of the cell itself. Infected cells, for instance, display information about specific antigens that managed to invade the cell. The information is very specific. It may read something like this:

"I have been invaded by a virus. Destroy me." *Or:*

"I have identified a foreign invader. More may be on the way. Alert the B cells to ready weapons." *Or:*

"I recognize the enemy. I am readying weapons to eliminate it." *Or:*

"I realize the body is threatened. I am dividing fast so that there are more of me."

Cell receptors can also indicate that the cell is ready to accept a shipment of raw materials (glucose, amino acids, vitamins).

Many effective medications take advantage of cell receptors. For example, to multiply, cells require the vitamin folic acid, which fits into a special receptor on the cell's surface. Since methotrexate fits that same receptor, the drug is used as a decoy, thereby depriving the cell of folic acid. In the presence of methotrexate, cell division is markedly decreased. This in turn diminishes activity of the immune system.

Weaponry

The specialized cells of the immune system manufacture dozens of specific and nonspecific body chemicals, including lysozymes, leukotrienes, antibodies, and cytokines, whose function is to reestablish order. As a group, these substances are called immunomodulators. Unfortunately, many of these weapons misfire in the civil war characteristic of RA.

Initial Response of the Immune System

The world is a hostile place. Every creature is constantly threatened by infectious agents and other foreign antigens. As soon as an antigen penetrates the outer defenses, the body mounts a nonspecific response. The blood supply to the affected area increases. The walls of the capillaries supplying the site of the injury become more permeable, allowing white blood cells and soluble mediators of immunity to congregate at the site of the accident. All this activity feeds on itself. The area becomes red, swells, and hurts. This can be seen in the overlying skin as inflammation.

Neutrophils, monocytes/macrophages, eosinophils, and basophils are alerted, rush to the site of the skirmish, and try to contain the invaders. Both neutrophils and monocytes/macrophages attempt to physically eliminate the intruder by engulfing it. This process is referred to as *phagocytosis* (eaten by cells). Indeed, *macrophage* means "big eater." Once ingested by the macrophage, the antigen is chopped to pieces by cellular chemicals. Some part of this antigen is displayed on the surface of the macrophage so that it can be identified and presented to other cells of the immune system.

All this activity generates loads of immune mediators. Those produced by the macrophages include substances that enhance cell destruction, increase blood flow, stimulate cell division, and in general create havoc and generate debris that must be cleared away. This in turn stimulates the production of corrosive lysosomal enzymes known to fuel the chronic inflammation characteristic of all forms of arthritis. The deleterious effects of some of these inflammatory products can be suppressed, or mitigated, by various anti-inflammatory drugs: NSAIDS, corticosteroids, and the new COX-2 inhibitors. As every arthritis sufferer knows only too well, the anti-inflammatory agents suppress the inflammation temporarily; they do not alter the underlying disease mechanism.

Delayed Response of the Immune System

Once alerted, the immune system readies its later defenses, the lymphocytes. There are two principal types of lymphocytes: B lymphocytes (B cells) and T lymphocytes (T cells). Their initials refer to the way these cells evolve from the stem cells. The B cells (the B refers to bursa of Fabricius) mature in the lymph nodes; the T cells mature in the thymus.

B Lymphocytes

When properly stimulated, the B lymphocytes give rise to plasma cells. A plasma cell is a "factory" that produces antibodies against specific infectious agents. Nature devised an ingenious system by which various B cells are able to manufacture thousands of specific antibodies against thousands of different antigens. The pattern for a particular antibody is stored in the memory of the B cells and retrieved whenever necessary.

During the initial nonspecific immune response, the circulating cells of the immune system fingerprint the antigen and present the information to the lymphocytes. If the antigen is familiar, the "memory" B cell quickly reactivates production of the matching antibody, and the host (i.e., us) is not even aware of the skirmish. If the invader is unfamiliar, antibody production takes a few days to get underway, during which time the host may develop a fever and/or a rash, and may feel ill.

Antibodies are proteins, more specifically immunoglobulins, mostly belonging to the gamma globulin family (IgG) or macroglobulin family (IgM). As a rule, antibodies are a good thing. People suffering from autoimmune diseases, however, produce antibodies against their own tissues.

B lymphocytes, and their descendents, plasma cells, are programmed to make specific substances that "handcuff" and eliminate specific invaders such as a flu virus. Any substance that can trigger the B cells to generate such a specific substance is called an *antigen*. The substance made by the B cells is called an *antibody*. In Greek, *anti* means "against." Once a B cell has learned to make an antibody to a specific antigen, it can always make this particular antibody, and only this antibody. The cell membrane of this particular B cell will have a receptor that recognizes only this particular antigen. When needed, the B cell evolves into a plasma cell, which then manufactures large amounts of this particular antibody. When the macrophages encounter a new antigen, they bring it over to the B cells, which tool up to manufacture a new, specific antibody.

T Lymphocytes

The antibodies produced by the B cells overwhelm the antigens in the extracellular fluid. They are ineffective whenever an antigen manages to penetrate a cell. This is where the T cells come in. There are two principal T cells—helper T cells and killer T cells—their names adequately describing their function in safeguarding the integrity of the body. Some scientists have assigned the role of master cell to the helper T cell.

After a macrophage has gobbled up an antigen, it displays a piece of this unwelcome guest on its surface where it may be approached by a helper T cell. Taking the MHC markers into consideration, the helper T cell decides on a course of action: Should there be an increase in antibody-producing B cells or in the number of killer T cells? The killer T cell is ferocious. It attaches itself to the offending cell and most often kills it quickly. Suffice it to say that the war waged by killer T cells against anything they consider "nonself" is merciless. In transplant medicine, killer T cells rapidly destroy unprotected transplanted organs. In AIDS, killer T cells destroy a person's immune system. In juvenile diabetes, an autoimmune disease somewhat similar to RA, T cells destroy the cells in the pancreas that manufacture insulin. The role that T cells play in rheumatoid arthritis is not yet completely understood, but T cells are found in large numbers in the rheumatoid synovium.

Fortunately, scientists are learning to manipulate T-cell response. In aggressive cases of RA, rheumatologists do sometimes use cyclosporine, an immunosuppressant that targets T cells and is so powerful that it prevents the rejection of transplanted organs. When used for more

HELPER T CELLS

When a helper T cell is approached by a macrophage, it becomes activated and alerts the entire immune system. Depending on the circumstances, the helper T cell may boost the number of antibody-producing B cells or increase the number of killer T cells.

KILLER T CELLS

When alerted, a killer T cell binds to a receptor of the offending cell. Upon a signal from the helper T cell, it becomes activated, and, if appropriate, destroys the infected cell.

than a year, large doses of cyclosporine may cause kidney damage and hypertension. Though these problems are less likely to occur with the currently used lower doses of cyclosporine, fewer problems are encountered with methotrexate, azathioprine, and leflunomide, which also target the lymphocytes.

Before dismissing the T cells as a total nuisance, let us remember that they are essential to our health. T-cell vigilance probably eliminates most cancers before they gain a foothold.

Soluble Mediators of Immunity: The Weapons of the Immune System

Most actions of the immune system are facilitated by the soluble mediators of immunity. Since their overproduction, as well as their suppression during treatment, plays a crucial role in RA, let us examine a few relevant ones in detail (see also Table 5–1). The production of soluble mediators of immunity varies with the stage of the immune response. Some mediators are produced during the initial phase and some appear later.

C-reactive protein (CRP) is produced in large amounts during the acute phase of the infection. It is used as a measure of RA disease activity.

Complement is a cascade of about 20 serum proteins that are part of the inflammatory process, attracting and activating the phagocytes, and lysing (perforating) cell membranes. Complement plays a role in fueling the inflammation characteristic of RA.

The *cytokine network* is an extremely large, varied number of mostly macrophage- and T-cell-produced proteins that mastermind the communication between cells, activating some and stimulating others to divide and multiply. Cytokines of special interest in RA include:

◆   *Interferons.* Interferons are "good" mediators produced by some activated T-helper cells. These proteins increase the resistance of cells to infection.

◆   *Interleukins and growth factors.* They stimulate the division of specific cells of the immune system. Interleukin-1 has major pro-inflammatory activity.

◆   *Tumor necrosis factor (TNF).* TNFs are cytotoxic, meaning they kill cells. When first discovered, this group of cytokines was believed to participate in the killing of tumor cells. Subsequently, they were shown to have wide-ranging activities. In autoimmune diseases, TNFs

TABLE 5-1. Immune Modulators and Other Substances That Play a Key Role in Immunity and Inflammation

Antibodies: Also called immunoglobulins. These proteins manufactured by B plasma cells are able to hook up with specific antigens. The resulting antibody-antigen complexes are gobbled up by phagocytic cells. Under certain circumstances, as in autoimmune disease, the B plasma cells manufacture autoantibodies.

Antigen: Any substance that induces the B plasma cells to produce an antibody.

C-reactive protein (CRP): Produced in large amounts during the acute phase of an infectious/inflammatory process. Used to gauge inflammatory activity in RA.

Complement: A group of 20 or more proteins that enhance the localized immune response. In particular, complement promotes phagocytosis and increases blood flow.

Cytokines: A general term for a large group of immune mediators including:

◆ Interferons, which increase the resistance of cells to infection.
◆ Interleukins, of which there are at least 17 (IL-1 to IL-17), and which are produced by the T cells and macrophages. The interleukins have wide-ranging effects including promotion of cell division, growth factor activity, and activation of B and T cells.
◆ Tumor necrosis factor, a pro-inflammatory mediator.

Prostaglandins: These hormone-like substances regulate important physiological processes including kidney function, blood pressure, inflammation, and the release of gastric acid and stomach-coating mucus. The prostaglandins play an important role in the joint inflammation characteristic of arthritis.

seem to promote the proliferation of inflammatory cells. In RA, TNF-alpha promotes proteoglycan and collagen breakdown, decreases bone synthesis, and increases PGE2 production. The administration of TNF-alpha inhibitors, such as etanercept and remicade, is an extremely promising new therapy for RA. The TNF-alpha antagonists bind or work as decoys and trap TNF-alpha prior to its binding to cells and causing inflammation and tissue damage.

Telltale Products of the Immune System

C-Reactive Protein

In 1930, scientists identified CRP, a new protein produced during pneumococcal pneumonia. This protein was also present in other diseases associated with inflammation or tissue damage. Its concentration in blood proved to be a reliable indicator of the inflammatory activity of RA. The test is now routinely used to gauge the activity of the disease at any time and to evaluate the effectiveness of a particular antirheumatic drug. It is more reliable than erythrocyte sedimentation rate (ESR) and identifies changes more quickly.

Rheumatoid Factor

Like many others, Russell L. Cecil, an early, influential American rheumatologist, believed that RA was caused by a streptococcus bacterium. To prove his point and to facilitate the diagnosis of RA, Cecil devised two laboratory tests. Though the tests often correctly identified patients suffering from rheumatoid arthritis, they were not very reliable, and Cecil did not pursue the matter.

Eric Waaler, a Norwegian investigator, also believed RA was an infectious disease. Waaler showed that specially treated sheep red blood cells clumped when mixed with the serum (blood minus red cells) of persons suffering from RA. Such agglutination did not occur when the sheep red blood cells were mixed with serum from normal controls. This difference was attributed to the presence of a protein later called rheumatoid factor (RF). Waaler's test was extremely sensitive, remaining positive when the serum of people suffering from RA was diluted 5,000-fold or more with water. Waaler reported his findings at a medical congress held in New York in September 1939. At that particular congress, medical news was dwarfed by the announcement that Germany invaded Poland on September 1. World War II had begun. Waaler returned to his native Norway. In 1940, the Nazis occupied his homeland, and his scientific discoveries would have to wait until the end of the hostilities.

The next chapter involving RF was written in 1948 at Columbia Presbyterian Medical Center in New York, where Harry M. Rose and his laboratory technician, Elisabeth Pearce, were studying another infection caused by a ricketsial organism—a type of virus. It so happened that their test, like Eric Waaler's, involved sensitized sheep red blood cells. At one point, Ms. Pearce, who suffered from RA, used her own blood as a "normal" control. The next morning, she noted that her blood strongly agglutinated the sheep red blood cells. Ms. Pearce reported these surprising results to her own rheumatologist, Charles Ragan. Instead of shrugging off the information, Dr. Ragan gave Ms. Pearce serum samples of five unknown patients. Using the new test, Ms. Pearce correctly identified the three people suffering from RA. RF turned out to be an antibody directed against a patient's own immunoglobulins. Similar self-reacting antibodies to collagen, chondrocytes, and other normal tissue of the articular joint demonstrate that RA is an autoimmune disorder. Because these antibodies are directed against a person's own tissue, they are called autoantibodies.

The RF test is positive in 80 percent of people suffering from RA. Since it misses 20 percent of those who suffer from the disease, its absence does not rule out RA. Moreover, it has many false positives and can be found in patients with other diseases such as systemic lupus erythematosus. Nevertheless, it is a very helpful diagnostic tool and may help physicians to support a clinical diagnosis of RA.

INFLAMMATION

How Rheumatoid Arthritis Develops

In RA, for still unknown reasons, the immune system considers its own joint tissues foreign. Once aroused, the immune system mobilizes an army of white blood cells and attempts to rid the body of this foreign intruder. This alarm to an unknown antigen simply creates havoc. What was to have been a temporary skirmish turns into a chronic, embattled stalemate. The immune system stays on alert. The war machine it created for the emergency remains mobilized and the civil war continues.

To begin with, white blood cells migrate into the joint cavity. The synovium becomes inflamed and engorged with fluid, causing synovitis. Lymphocytes and macrophages continue to pour into the joint cavity, where they multiply, differentiate, and release their cargo of inflammatory mediators: cytokines, leukotrienes, prostaglandins, and so forth. Some of these stimulate the growth of blood vessels, which in turn supply the growing cell mass with nutrients. Within weeks or months after the inflammatory process has started, the synovium has become thickened.

As the disease progresses, the cells take up permanent residence, forming a pannus (Fig. 5-1). In Latin, *pannus* means "a piece of cloth." In RA, it refers to the mass of synovial tissue that spreads over the top of cartilage in a rheumatoid joint. Typically, a pannus is a mass of white blood cells: macrophages, fibroblasts, T cells, B cells, neutrophils, natural killer cells, helper cells, phagocytes, lymphocytes, and others. These cells produce rheumatoid factor, other immune complexes, prostaglandins, cytokines, and the other mediators discussed in this chapter.

FIGURE 5-1. **Formation of a Pannus.** A schematic view of the events occurring in an inflamed synovial joint. Pro-inflammatory cytokines initiate the pile-up of inflammatory cells and debris (pannus) in a rheumatoid joint. Note the growing pannus in the left lower corner of the synovial space that is spreading across the entire joint surface. *Drawing courtesy of Amgen Inc.*

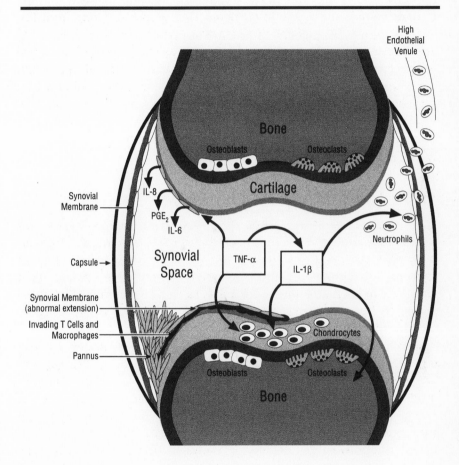

These chemicals self-perpetuate the rheumatoid disease process. A rheumatoid synovium is so busy producing these chemicals that it can be compared to a lymph node whose function is to participate in the overall immune response and therefore produce quantities of immune modulators.

Currently, scientists are busy sorting out both the cells that are present in the rheumatoid synovium and the substances produced by these cells. As these facts become more clearly understood, the treatment of

RA will improve. Chapters 7, 8, and 9 review the medications currently used in the treatment of RA. All interrupt one or more of the inflammatory pathways. At present, these blockades are rather clumsy because they also interrupt useful body functions. As our understanding of RA grows, scientists may find ways of interrupting these pathways more accurately.

◆ CHAPTER ◆

6

Drugs, Drugs, and More Drugs

To a large extent, new and powerful medications are responsible for the elimination of killer diseases, the increase in life expectancy, and improved overall health. This chapter reviews some general facts about drugs and drug therapy.

Most people who hear the word *arthritis* think "pain medication." Indeed, patients suffering from arthritis are a boon to the drug industry. Each year, doctors write millions of prescriptions for antiarthritis drugs, netting the industry over $2 billion. In 1992, an additional billion was spent on non-prescription painkillers such as aspirin, acetaminophen, and ibuprofen. You will need more than painkillers to keep your RA in check. Fifty or more different drugs are commonly used in the management of RA.

The availability of many drugs is largely responsible for our better health. To quote Dr. Victor R. Fuchs, a leading medical ethicist, "The great power of drugs is a development of the 20th century. Our age has been given many names—atomic, electronic, space, and the like—but measured by the impact on people's lives, it might just as well be called the drug age."

Most of these drugs are powerful. Taking medications properly is an important aspect of your self-care. According to the *Journal of the American Medical Association* (January 21, 1996), in a study of admissions to leading Boston hospitals it was estimated that 6.5 percent were due to adverse drug reactions or an unfortunate combination of drugs. Often, these hospitalizations are not due to carelessness but to reactions to powerful drugs prescribed for desperately ill patients. In order to minimize mishaps, discuss newly prescribed drugs with your doctor.

HOW TO TALK ABOUT DRUGS

Every field has its own special vocabulary with which we must be familiar to feel at home. Music lovers talk of beats, half-notes, scales, sharps, and flats; baseball fans of home runs, batters, pitchers, and outfielders; doctors of concomitant disease, X rays, imaging, and exclusion. So it is with drugs. Your doctor or pharmacist may talk about generic equivalents, trade names, over-the-counter (OTC) agents, or experimental drugs.

In general, all drugs have a *chemical name* that describes their chemical nature. The chemical name for aspirin is acetylsalicylic acid; the chemical name for Plaquenil is 2-[[4-[(7-chloro-4-quinolyl)amino]pentyl]-ethylamino]ethanol sulfate. All drugs have a *generic (common) name.* Auranofin is the common name for oral gold. Piroxicam is the generic name for Feldene.

The drug's *trade* or *brand name* is the name given to it by the pharmaceutical company that developed or manufactures the drug. Feldene is Pfizer's name for piroxicam. Aspirin, now a household word, is the original trade name for acetylsalicylic acid developed by Bayer.

At first, all newly developed drugs are proprietary and patented and are sold by the drug company that developed them. These drugs are usually expensive because there is no competition. Also, some drugs are expensive to manufacture. Furthermore, the market for the medication may be small.

After a number of years, the patent protecting the drug runs out and other drug companies can manufacture the same drug. These drugs, referred to as *generic equivalents,* are usually cheaper. Some companies create their own trade names for generic equivalents.

Many of the drugs used for the treatment of RA are generic because they have been around for a long time, including gold, hydroxychloroquine, acetylsalicylic acid, acetaminophen, and prednisone.

Prescription and Nonprescription Drugs

Drugs are either prescription drugs or nonprescription (over the counter or OTC) drugs. The idea behind a nonprescription drug is that it is usually safe enough to take without the supervision of a physician. This, however, is not always the case. Aspirin, which is still a major drug for the treatment of RA, is an OTC drug, as is acetaminophen (Tylenol). Both are strong medications, and, as is discussed in the next chapter, they were discovered long before there were any agencies regulating their safe use.

Your Pharmacist

In the olden days when pharmacists gathered herbs and prepared medications, they were indispensable members of the health care team. Today, most medications are prepared in big factories.

Pharmacists are highly skilled professionals who are able to identify potential drug interactions. Some pharmacies keep drug profiles (lists) of the drugs taken by their regular clients. This is important because many of us consult several doctors, each of whom might prescribe a different medication.

If you buy all your drugs at the same pharmacy, the pharmacist may alert the doctor if your newly prescribed medication—for example, an antibiotic or a sleeping pill—could interfere with a drug that you are already taking.

Drug-Drug Interactions

Most RA patients take more than one drug, and these drugs can interfere with one another in many different ways. Here are a few examples:

◆ Two drugs that have the same effect enhance each other, and the combined effect may be excessive. An example is aspirin, which has some anticoagulant properties, in combination with an anticoagulant such as Coumadin. Two medications that depress the central nervous system, such as a sleeping pill and a tranquilizer, are another example.

◆ Drugs may have opposite effects and cancel each other out, for example, Coumadin and vitamin K. Coumadin increases the time it takes blood to coagulate and therefore reduces the tendency to form a thrombus, whereas vitamin K is an essential part of the blood coagulation process and speeds it up. The drugs cancel each other out because Coumadin actually inhibits the formation of vitamin K-related clotting factors. Sometimes this opposing effect is useful, for example, vitamin K is used as an antidote for Coumadin overdosage.

◆ Sometimes one drug reduces or enhances the absorption of a drug from the gastrointestinal tract. Antacids, for example, reduce the absorption of aspirin from the stomach. Laxatives, which speed up the rate at which food travels through the gut, often decrease drug absorption.

Fortunately, these drug interactions are taken into account when prescribing medications. Some of them are overcome by staggering when the medications are taken. Sometimes, the dose of one or both medications is increased or decreased. In any case, it is necessary to check with your doctor and pharmacist on how, why, and when to take your medication.

Drug-Nutrient Interactions

Drugs can affect the way your body utilizes foods. Mineral oil, for instance, coats the intestine, thereby interfering with the absorption of some vitamins and drugs, such as the NSAIDs, which must be taken with food to protect the lining of the stomach. For more details, see Chapter 11.

Dosage

When developing a new drug, the pharmaceutical manufacturer carefully evaluates the correct balance between *absorption* and *elimination*. The resulting information is translated into *dosage* (the amount of drug taken or injected) and *frequency of administration*.

Some drugs are eliminated quickly and must be taken quite often. Aspirin, for example, has a $t^1/2$ of 30 minutes. For the blood level to remain above the minimal effective serum level, it should be taken every 4 hours. Some of the newer nonsteroidal anti-inflammatory drugs (NSAIDs) are eliminated more slowly, and therefore need to be taken only once or twice a day.

The following considerations are taken into account when determining the dosage schedule:

◆ *Input:* When taken orally (by mouth), most drugs are absorbed rapidly into the blood, within 15 minutes to 2 hours. Drugs can be formulated so that they are released more slowly over a longer period of time (sustained release). When injected intravenously, the entire dose reaches the blood immediately.

◆ *Output:* The body considers all drugs (medications and social drugs such as alcohol) poisons to be gotten rid of as quickly as possible. The speed at which this occurs is called the *rate of elimination*. This rate is expressed as $t^1/2$, or the time, in minutes or hours, it takes the body to get rid of half the administered amount of drug.

◆ *Minimum effective serum level:* To do its job, the drug must be present in the blood at a specific level known as the minimum effective serum level. For example, if you take one Tylenol instead of two, the drug may not alleviate your pain. Giving more than the required amount of drug is useless and perhaps even harmful. The rate of absorption and elimination of two drugs is shown in Figure 6–1. Note that drug B never reaches its minimum effective level in the blood.

What to Ask About Any Newly Prescribed Drug

◆ What is the name of the drug?

◆ Does the drug have a (cheaper) generic equivalent?

◆ How often should I take the medication?

◆ How much should I take?

◆ When should I take the medication?

◆ Should I take the medication with food or on an empty stomach (1 hour before meals or 2 hours after meals)?

◆ How long should I take the medication for?

◆ Should the prescription be refilled if it runs out before my next appointment?

◆ What should I do if I forget to take the medication?

FIGURE 6-1. **Absorption and Elimination of a Drug.** After 3 hours, the amount of drug A has fallen below its minimum effective level. In order to maintain the minimum effective level in the blood, the patient must take another does at the time specified by the drug manufacturer.

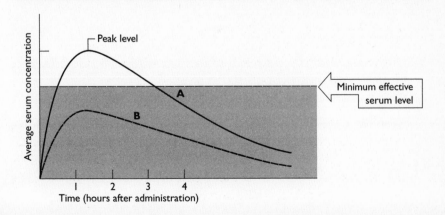

◆ What side effects does the medication have? Does it produce stomach upset, stomach irritation, sleepiness, or other side effects?

◆ Will the medication make me less alert when driving or operating dangerous machinery?

◆ Will it affect my menstrual period?

◆ Does the medication have to be discontinued if I plan to become pregnant?

◆ Will drinking beer, wine, or liquor interfere with my medication?

◆ Will the medication interfere with sleep?

◆ Does the medication interfere with nonprescription drugs such as aspirin, allergy pills, laxatives, or others?

◆ Is there anything else special about this medication?

THE GAME PLAN FOR RA

Five major classes of drugs are used for the treatment of RA:

1. Nonsteroidal anti-inflammatory drugs (NSAIDs) and analgesics (Chapter 7)
2. Disease-modifying antirheumatic drugs (DMARDs; Chapter 8)
3. Corticosteroids (Chapter 9)
4. Immunosuppressives (Chapter 8)
5. Biologics (Chapter 8)

Chapter 5 explored reasons why some of these medications may be effective for the treatment of RA.

In addition to the medications to control RA, the following medications are often prescribed:

1. Stronger analgesics (painkillers) to reduce pain
2. Drugs to protect the stomach from gastrointestinal side effects of NSAIDs and corticosteroids (Chapter 7)
3. Drugs to prevent corticosteroid-induced osteoporosis (bone loss; Chapter 9)

Chapters 7, 8, and 9 deal with the principal classes of drugs used to manage RA.

◆ CHAPTER ◆

7

Aspirin, Other Nonsteroidal Anti-Inflammatory Drugs, Super-Aspirins, and Other Analgesics

---◦◉◦---

The chapter provides information about the history and mode of action of aspirin, other NSAIDs, super-aspirin (COX-2), and other anti-inflammatories.

Most of the painkillers used in the management of RA are nonsteroidal anti-inflammatory drugs (NSAIDS). These medications decrease pain and inflammation, but they are not steroids like prednisone and its relatives. For a very long time, aspirin, the best known NSAID, was the only effective medication for all forms of arthritis. Occasionally, the NSAIDs are referred to as fast-acting antiarthritis drugs to differentiate them from the slower-acting drugs considered in the next chapter.

ASPIRIN: THE FIRST MIRACLE DRUG

Plant extracts containing salicylic acid (from *salix,* Latin for "willow"), a chemical substance, were used in ancient Egypt and in Rome to calm fever and pain. Similar preparations were widely used in England during the

18th century. In 1758, Reverend Edward Stone tested this folk remedy in an early drug trial. Stone made a willow bark extract and prescribed it to 50 patients suffering from a variety of painful and/or feverish ailments. The potion indeed reduced pain and fever. Five years later, Reverend Stone reported his experiment to the Royal Society in London, then the world's most revered scientific organization. Soon thereafter, an Italian chemist discovered that the painkilling properties of the extract were due to salicylic acid, a chemical component of the bark.

The use of the drug was limited because salicylic acid irritated the stomach. During the 1850s, Felix Hofman, a chemist employed by Bayer Pharmaceuticals in Germany, searched the literature for a gentler pain-relieving drug. Hofman came across a scientific report indicating that in 1853 Charles Fredrick von Gerhart, a French chemist, had prepared acetylsalicylic acid, a drug that retained the desirable properties of sali-cylic acid, but was less irritating to the stomach. Hofman called the drug *Aspirin* and was overjoyed when it eased the pain of his severely arthritic father. Aspirin soon became the most widely used drug in the world.

Aspirin is a true miracle drug. For more than a century, it has low-ered fever, alleviated pain, and suppressed the inflammation character-istic of many forms of arthritis. Aspirin is a powerful drug. The fact that it is available without prescription is an accident of its birth.

NEWER NSAIDS

Aspirin reigned supreme for a century. It is a very potent drug, and still is the gold standard against which all comparable medications are mea-sured. Aspirin also has the marked advantage of being inexpensive. Dur-ing the 1950s, Merck developed indomethacin (Indocin), which worked like aspirin, but was thought to have fewer gastric side effects. Since then, two dozen similar drugs have appeared on the market. They suppress fever, pain, and inflammation; however, they differ from one another suf-ficiently with respect to side effects, onset and duration of action, and patient response. To find the one that is best for you is usually a matter of trial and error. Table 7-1 lists commonly prescribed NSAIDs, dosage, and length of action.

Most drugs listed in Table 7-1 are prescription drugs. A few (ibupro-fen, indomethacin, naproxen) are also available over the counter. Be aware that an OTC preparation usually contains less drug than the pre-scription version.

TABLE 7-1. Nonsteroidal Anti-inflammatory Drugs

Generic Name*	Trade Name†	$t^{1}/_2$‡	Form/Dosage	Remarks
Acetylsalicylic acid	Aspirin	0.5	Tablets: 325, 500, 600, 650 mg	Available without prescription under many different names.
Diclofenac	Voltaren	1–2	Tablets: 25, 50, 75 mg	Tablets are enteric coated.
Diflusinal	Dolobid	8–12	Tablets: 250, 500 mg	The drug is a salicylate-like aspirin.
Etodolac	Lodine	7–8	Capsules: 200, 300 mg	
Fenoprofen	Nalfon	3	Capsules: 200, 300 mg Tablets: 600 mg	Not for patients with kidney disease.
Flurbiprofen	Ansaid	6	Tablets: 50, 100 mg	Maximum dose 300 mg/day.
Ibuprofen	Motrin Advil Nuprin	2 2 2	Tablets: 300, 400, 600, 800 mg	This drug is available without prescription. All OTC preparations contain 200 mg/tablet. OTC trade names include Advil, Ibiprin, Ibu-Tab, Menadol, Midol, Nuprin, and others.
Indomethacin	Indocin	5	Capsules: 25, 50 mg Rectal suppositories: 50 mg Capsules: 75 mg	
	Indocin SR	5		
Ketorolac	Acolar, Toradol	4–6	Tablets: 10 mg	Available as intramuscular injection.

(continued)

TABLE 7-1. *(continued)*

Generic Name*	Trade Name†	$t^{1/2}$‡	Form/Dosage	Remarks
Ketoprofen	Orudis	2–5	Tablets: 25 mg	Use reduced dosage for patients with kidney disease.
Meclofenamate	Heclofen, Meclomen	2–3	Tablets: 50, 100 mg	
Mefenamic acid	Ponstel	2–4	Capsules: 250 mg	Use 1 week only.
Mesalamine	Asacol	0.5–1.5	Rectal suppositories: 500 mg Suspensions: 4g/60 mL Delayed-release tablets: 800 mg	Counterindicated for patients with sensitivity to sulfite.
Meloxicam	Mobic	1	Tablets: 7.5 mg	Long half-life
Nabumetone	Relafen	22–30	Tablets: 500, 750 mg	
Naproxen	Naprosyn	12–15	Tablets: 250, 375, 500 mg	This drug is available without prescription. All OTC preparations contain 200 mg/ tablet.
Naproxen sodium	Anaprox Aleve	12–15	Tablets: 250, 375, 500 mg	
Oxaprozin	Daypro	20–25	Capsules: 600 mg	
Piroxicam	Feldene	50	Capsules: 10, 20 mg	Note that this drug is exceedingly long-lasting (long half-life.)
Sulindac	Clinoril	8	Tablets: 150, 200 mg	
Tolmetin	Tolectin	1	Tablets: 400 mg Capsules: 400 mg	

*The generic name is the common name of the drug.
†The trade name, also called the proprietary name, is the name given to the drug by the manufacturer. Most of the drugs listed are available in Canada, sometimes under a different name.
‡$t^{1/2}$ is the time it takes for half of the drug to be eliminated from the body. It means that it takes a short half hour for the body to get rid of half an aspirin tablet and 50 hours to get rid of half a Feldene tablet. To maintain an effective minimum dose (see Chapter 6), you must take aspirin every 4 hours and Feldene only once a day.

Source: Information from *The Nurse's Drug Handbook*, 7th ed., by Suzanne Loebl, George Spratto, and Adrienne Woods (1994). Delmar Publishers Inc., Albany, NY.

Two regular (325 mg/tablet) aspirin or one arthritis-strength (500 mg/tablet) aspirins taken every 4 hours should provide pain relief. A much larger dose is required when the drug is used to suppress inflammation. Put differently, the minimal effective anti-inflammatory level is higher than the minimal effective analgesic level.

How to Take NSAIDs

Gastrointestinal irritation (heartburn, ulcers, dyspepsia, nausea, vomiting) is the most common side effect of NSAIDs. The extent of the discomfort varies, but for many patients the benefits of the drugs outweigh the disadvantages. Table 7-2 suggests ways of decreasing gastrointestinal irritation caused by NSAIDs. It is also possible to diminish gastrointestinal irritation by protecting the gastric mucosa with an additional medication. Table 7-3 lists commonly employed medications. Table 7-4 lists side effects of NSAIDs and COX-2 inhibitors.

Table 7-2. Decreasing the Gastric Irritation Caused by NSAIDs

- Always take NSAIDs with food or soon after a meal.
- Avoid consuming other stomach irritants such as caffeine-containing beverages (coffee, tea, colas), alcohol, or chocolate.
- Select an agent that you can tolerate. Aspirin is particularly irritating. Some of the newer NSAIDs are easier on the stomach.
- Use enteric-coated medications that only release their drug in the small intestine, thereby protecting the gastric mucosa (lining of the stomach).

Table 7-3. Drugs Used to Protect the Intestinal Mucosa

- H-2 blockers such as cimetidine (Tagamet) and ranitidine (Zantac); proton-pump inhibitors such as omeprazole (Prilosec) and lansoprozole (Prevacid). These agents inhibit the release of gastric acid.
- Misoprostol (Cytotec), a synthetic prostaglandin, is able to stimulate the lining of the stomach to produce its protective mucus.
- Sucralfate (Carafate), a coating agent, protects ulcer sites and promotes healing by eliminating additional irritation of the wound.
- Antacids such as Rolaids, Tums, milk of magnesia, Mylanta, Alka-Seltzer, and others alleviate the stomach's excess acidity. Aspirin preparations premixed with antacids (buffered aspirin) are widely available.

TABLE 7-4. Side Effects of NSAIDs and COX-2 Inhibitors

- *Allergy:* An allergy to any of these agents requires immediate discontinuation. Allergy may develop after years of symptom-free usage. Allergic symptoms include acute asthma, skin rash, and nasal discharge.

- *Gastrointestinal problems:* These very common side effects range from mild discomfort and heartburn to intestinal and gastric ulceration and bleeding.

- *Blood coagulation:* Most of the agents slow blood coagulation. (The COX-2 inhibitors do not.) This is why the drugs must be discontinued weeks before elective surgery.

- *Rarely occurring side effects:* Dizziness, drowsiness, mental confusion, depression, other central nervous system effects, ringing in the ears, alteration of kidney function. People suffering from diabetes may find that the drugs lower blood sugar. This may require adjustment of insulin medication.

HOW TO READ THE LABEL OF NONPRESCRIPTION DRUGS

We are all familiar with food labels and with the information they provide. Nonprescription medication must have labels that list the nature of the drug, the amount of drug each pill contains, and other pertinent information. Table 7–5 explains how to read the label of an OTC preparation. The exact wording and the order in which the information is shown vary.

HOW ASPIRIN AND OTHER NSAIDS WORK

Aspirin has four different effects:

1. It lowers fever.
2. It decreases pain.
3. It decreases inflammation.
4. It is a mild anticoagulant (prevents blood clotting).

The discovery of how aspirin accomplishes these feats earned J. R. Vane part of the 1982 Nobel prize for medicine, the greatest honor that can be bestowed upon an investigator.

TABLE 7-5. How to Read the Label of an OTC Painkiller

Special message	May indicate some advantage of the product, such as "arthritis strength," "extra strength," "sustained release,"* or "enteric coated."†
Active ingredients	The ingredient portion of the label includes the chemical name of the active drug(s) in the preparation such as acetylsalicylic acid, acetaminophen, caffeine,‡ antacids, and so on. For preparations containing more than one active ingredient, the agents are listed in descending order, by weight.
Inactive ingredients	Starch, stearic acid, silicone, or other inert substances used to make the tablet or capsule.
Indications	The purpose for which the medication is to be taken, such as temporary relief of minor aches and pains, headaches, and fever.
Warning	Explains risks. For example: Keep out of reach of children. Do not use without doctor's orders. Do not use during pregnancy.
Dosage	Suggestions about amount of drug to be taken.

*The drug is released over a period of time. In this way, a drug with a short $t^{1/2}$ lasts longer.
†The tablet is coated and only releases its drug cargo in the small intestine, not in the stomach.
‡Caffeine is believed to enhance the effectiveness of some drugs.

Source: From *The Columbia Presbyterian Osteoarthritis Handbook.* R.P. Grelsemar and S. Loebl, eds., Macmillan, 1996. Reproduced with permission.

The first prostaglandin was discovered in the prostate gland (hence its name) in 1923 by Ulf von Euler. Close to two dozen different prostaglandins are known today.

It turned out that these short-lived hormone-like substances regulate many normal body functions: blood flow, blood coagulation, kidney function, and the secretion of mucus by the lining of the stomach. Inflammation and pain, which are the body's healthy response to injury, are also masterminded by prostaglandins.

All prostaglandins originate from a substance called *arachidonic acid,* which is part of the thin membrane that encloses each cell. In living organisms the transformation of one substance into another proceeds in stepwise fashion, each small step being carried out by a specific enzyme. Thus, the formation of prostaglandins from arachidonic acid and the transformation of one prostaglandin into another is carried out by specific enzymes (see Table 7–6).

The NSAIDS are able to interrupt this prostaglandin cascade by "knocking out" enzymes called COX-1 and COX-2, which mastermind the transformation of arachidonic acid into prostaglandins. Unfortunately, this curtails the production of all prostaglandins, including those that carry out the body's housekeeping functions such as the production of the mucus that coats the stomach, as well as those that promote pain and inflammation. This is why aspirin has so many unpleasant side effects.

TABLE 7-6. How Aspirin, Other Nonsteroidal Anti-inflammatories, and COX-2 Work

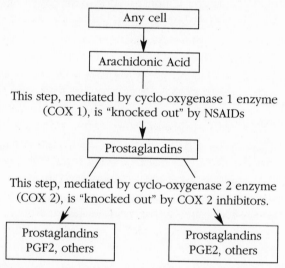

These prostaglandins regulate the function of the platelets, kidney, and the integrity of the stomach lining.

These prostaglandins stimulate the immune system and fuel inflammation.

Prostaglandin cascade: Prostaglandins (PG), formed from arachidonic acid in the cell membrane, are hormone-like substances that participate in major biological processes. The transformation of one PG into another requires specific enzymes, among them COX-1 and COX-2. The NSAIDs "knock out" COX-1, thereby halting the entire PG cascade. COX-2 interrupts the PG cascade after it splits into the "good" PGs (PGF2, thromboxane), which participate in essential housekeeping tasks such as protecting the lining of the stomach, kidney function, and blood coagulation, and into the "bad" PGs (PGE2, others), which stimulate the immune system and fuel inflammation. This is why COX-2 inhibitors such as celecoxib (Celebrex) are easier on the stomach.

COX-2 INHIBITORS

As previously explained, the raw material for the production of prosta-glandins is arachidonic acid, which is part of the cell membrane. An enzyme called cyclo-oxygenase transforms arachidonic acid into prostaglandins, which then undergo other changes. Moreover, the chronic inflammation characteristic of arthritis stimulates the production of inflammation-causing prostaglandins, especially PGE2. Corticosteroids and large doses of NSAIDs can halt this transformation, but as previously discussed, the drugs also prevent the formation of the good prostaglandins involved in housekeeping functions.

A close look at the mechanism of action of the NSAIDs in the early 1990s convinced Philip Needleman, a pharmaceutical chemist, that two separate enzymes were involved in the process: COX-1, which leads to the formation of a common prostaglandin precursor; and COX-2, which is more specifically involved in the genesis of the inflammatory prostaglandin cascade.

Further investigation supported Needleman's hunches, and he concentrated on discovering a drug that would selectively block the COX-2 enzyme. Years of research paid off, and COX-2 inhibitors are now available (Table 7-7). Since these agents interrupt the prostaglandin cascade at a latex branch, they do not interfere with the housekeeping functions of the prostaglandins; they may become the arthritis sufferer's new best friend. It will take time for doctors and patients to become used to these new drugs. Unknown side effects may appear down the road. Remember that aspirin has been with us for 125 years! In many patients, COX-2 inhibitors have fewer gastrointestinal side effects than traditional NSAIDs (see Table 7–4).

TABLE 7-7. COX-2 Inhibitors

Generic Name	Trade Name	$t^{1/2}$	Form/Dosage
Celecoxib	Celebrex	11	Capsules: 100 mg Recommended dosage: 100–200 mg twice a day
Rofecoxib	Vioxx	17	Tablets: 12.5 mg Oral suspension: 12.5 mg/5 mL Recommended dosage: Initially 12.5 mg/day, then 25 mg/day when indicated

OTHER ANALGESICS

The NSAIDs relieve pain and inflammation. Arthritis patients, however, also utilize medications that only relieve pain. The ones most commonly used are discussed next.

Acetaminophen

Acetaminophen (Anacin, Exedrin, Tylenol, others) is almost as well known and as old as aspirin. Like aspirin, it is inexpensive and available without prescription. Also like aspirin, the drug lowers pain and fever, but it has no anti-inflammatory effect.

The drug acts primarily via the central nervous system and does not interfere with prostaglandin production. Therefore, it does not irritate the stomach. Serious side effects (liver and kidney damage) may occur after prolonged usage.

Acetaminophen comes in different strengths: regular strength (325 mg), extra or arthritis strength (500 mg), and slow release (650 mg). Acetaminophen is sometimes mixed with other agents. The most common of these are antihistamines, which induce sleep and relieve sinus congestion, and caffeine, which is supposed to enhance its pain-relieving effects.

Dosage: 3–4 g/day.

Codeine

Codeine is a morphine-type narcotic analgesic. It is minimally addictive. Codeine is an effective cough suppressant and an excellent analgesic. It is a powerful central nervous system (CNS) suppressant. When prescribed for pain, it is usually mixed with acetaminophen or aspirin. Side effects include dizziness, drowsiness, nausea, vomiting, and constipation. Other CNS depressants (alcohol, sleeping pills, antianxiety and antipsychotic agents) should be used with caution or not at all.

Dosage: 15–60 mg/day.

Propoxyphene Hydrochloride

These nonnarcotic analgesics (e.g., Darvon, Wygesic) relieve pain by depressing the CNS. Prolonged use may prove to be addictive. Side effects include nausea, vomiting, and dizziness. Depression (current or previous) is a contraindication. Other CNS depressants (alcohol, sleeping pills, antianxiety and antipsychotic agents) should be used with caution or not at all.

Tramadol

Tramadol (Ultram) is effective for moderate to severe pain. It acts via the CNS, binding to opioid receptors. The drug is much less potent than morphine. Side effects include nausea, vomiting, dizziness/vertigo, headache, itching, dry mouth, and constipation. To minimize these side effects, your doctor may advise you to start with a lower dosage and increase it slowly until you reach the full dose.

Narcotic Analgesics

The narcotic analgesics, which include opium, morphine, codeine, and their relatives, have been around since the dawn of history. They are excellent painkillers, but since they are addictive, physicians were reluctant to prescribe them. However, this attitude is changing, and today these agents are prescribed more readily. The drugs act via the CNS, attaching to the opioid receptors, altering pain perception, and, at higher doses, creating euphoria. Side effects include respiratory depression, dizziness, sedation, headache, nausea, and vomiting. Frequently prescribed narcotic analgesics include oxycodone (Vicodin, Percocet, Duragesic, OxyContin) and morphine.

Tricyclic Antidepressants

Tricyclic antidepressants (amitriptyline, doxepin, nortriptyline), which block central pain receptors, are sometimes used in conjunction with pain medication. Side effects include sedation, confusion, anxiety, depression, and headache.

Topical Agents

Creams and lotions are widely advertised as providing pain relief. For patients suffering from RA, most pain originates so deeply within the body that it cannot be relieved by topical applications of ointments. There is, however, no harm in trying. As a general rule, topical agents are more effective for dull pain than sharp pain.

Topical creams either provide local analgesia or work as counterirritants. The latter stimulate nerve endings in the skin, inducing cold, warmth, numbing, itching, or other sensations that distract awareness from the primary pain. Counterirritants commonly contain camphor, menthol, histamine dihydrochloride, ammonia, methyl salicylate, and/or turpentine oils.

These topical agents should only be applied to intact skin. Because they are irritating, they must be kept away from the eyes. They are for external use only and should never be taken by mouth.

8

Disease-Modifying Antirheumatic Drugs (DMARDs)

This chapter is an in-depth review of the second-line agents used in the management of rheumatoid arthritis.

Once you have received a definite diagnosis of RA, it is likely that your doctor will prescribe one or several of a group of drugs that slow or stop joint damage and cause your disease to go into remission. A remission means that all, most, or many of the symptoms of your RA disappear. Blood test abnormalities may or may not improve.

According to the American College of Rheumatology (ACR), a patient is in remission when two or more of the following occur for at least 2 consecutive months:

1. Morning stiffness of 15 minutes or less

2. No fatigue

3. No joint pain

4. No joint tenderness

5. No swelling of the soft tissues (joints or tendon sheaths)

6. An erythrocyte sedimentation rate (ESR)[1] rate of 30 mm/hr (women) or 20 mm/hr (men)

7. Absence of systemic complications of RA

Remissions can occur spontaneously, but most often they are medication induced.

TERMINOLOGY

The group of drugs used to achieve remission goes by several names. This is in itself an indication that none of the designations is perfect:

Remitting drugs: Since the remission induced by these drugs is rarely long term, this name is outdated.

Disease-modifying antirheumatic drugs (DMARDs): This name is criticized because it is not understood how these agents modify RA.

Slow-acting antirheumatic drugs (SAARDs): This name is also imprecise because the beneficial effect of some members of the group (e.g., methotrexate) appears quite rapidly.

Second-line therapies: This again is an imprecise term because currently therapy with this group of drugs is usually initiated soon after RA has been diagnosed.

To avoid confusion, the term *DMARDs* is used throughout this book.

INITIATION OF DMARD THERAPY

The use of medications that induce remissions in RA is not new. Until recently, gold was the most commonly administered DMARD, and it was first used during the 1920s. What is new and important, however, is that these drugs are now used early in the course of RA. Indeed, on its Web page, the American College of Rheumatology (ACR) declares, "Using DMARDS [soon after a definite diagnosis has been made] represents a major change in the approach to the treatment of RA."

---

[1]This laboratory test is a measure of systemic inflammation. It is increased when the RA is active.

This new approach is successful. When physicians compared the joint damage of patients who received DMARDs as soon as the disease was diagnosed with patients who received these drugs 6 to 9 months later, there was no doubt that early, aggressive treatment paid off handsomely. In addition, this approach also prevents or reduces systemic manifestations of RA.

Once rheumatologists decided that it was important to treat RA early in its course, they hoped that they might achieve their goal more easily if they used more than one powerful agent. Today, many patients are often treated with a combination of DMARDs or DMARDs in combination with corticosteroids.

GOLD: THE FIRST DMARD

Since most DMARDs were discovered by accident, it is of interest to recall how gold came to be used in rheumatology. Seventy-five years ago, physicians believed that arthritis was caused by an infectious agent akin to the one causing tuberculosis. At the time, gold was used to treat tuberculosis, and Jacques Forrestier, a young French physician, decided to try intramuscular injections of a gold compound for his RA patients. The patients did not improve and Forrestier was ready to abandon the treatment. When Jacques Forrestier's father, also a physician, heard that his son was about to give up on gold, he muttered something about the impatience of young people. To humor his father, young Forrestier persisted with his gold injections. After 6 months or so, 70 to 80 percent of his RA patients improved even though the reason for using the drug was based on two false assumptions: Gold does not cure tuberculosis and RA is not an infectious disease. Ever since that time, gold injections have enabled tens of thousands of arthritis patients to lead productive, relatively pain-free lives. Even today, it is not really known how gold works.

TODAY'S DMARDS

Often, when there are multiple choices for the treatment of a specific disease, none is perfect. RA is a case in point. Its management is a matter of trial and error. Table 8–1 lists DMARDs currently used for the treatment of RA.

TABLE 8-1. DMARDs Used for the Treatment of RA

Cytotoxic Agents	Miscellaneous Agents
Azathioprine (Imuran)	Auranofin (Ridaura)
Cyclophosphamide (Cytoxan, others)	Aurothioglucose (Solganal)
Cyclosporine (Neoral, Sandimmune)	Gold sodium thiomalate (Myochrysine)
Leflunomide (Arava)	Hydroxychloroquine (Plaquenil, others)
Methotrexate (Rheumatrex, others)	Minocycline (Minocin)
Immunomodulators	D-penicillamine (Cuprimine, Depen)
Etanercept (Enbrel)	Sulfasalazine (Azulfidine, Sulfasalazine, others)
Infliximab (Remicade)	

Even a superficial glance at the list reveals that these drugs represent a curious mixture. They include:

◆ Gold, a precious metal

◆ D-penicillamine, a waste product of the manufacture of penicillin

◆ Hydroxychloroquine (Plaquenil), an antimalarial

◆ Methotrexate, an antimetabolite inherited from cancer therapy

◆ Cyclosporine, an immunosuppressant used in transplantation medicine

◆ Sulfasalazine, one of the very few drugs specifically developed to treat RA, but until recently used most often in the management of ulcerative colitis

◆ Etanercept, a tumor necrosis factor antagonist

The understanding of RA is growing rapidly. Within the next decade, the mode of action of these agents may be clarified and physicians will be able to select the one ideally suited for each patient.

All patients suffering from serious, chronic disease owe a debt of gratitude to the powerful medications physicians can use in their treatment. Patients with heart disease survive because of antihypertensives, antiarrhythmics, and vasodilators. Some cancers have become curable, and immunosuppressive agents permit people to tolerate donated organs. The treatment of RA is no exception.

Most riches have a dark side. Powerful medications usually have serious side effects. In most cases, this does not preclude their use. It simply means that you and your doctor will have to be alert to these side effects and change your medication schedule should they become dangerous. Your doctor will monitor you as often as necessary and teach you how to identify major side effects should they occur.

The dosage, side effects, and other important facts of currently used DMARDs are reviewed next. The drugs are arranged as shown in Table 8-1.

General Precautions for People Taking DMARD Medication

◆ Be sure to inform all your health care providers of the medications you are taking.

◆ Many of these medications suppress the immune system and increase your susceptibility to infections. Your reduced resistance may interfere with routine vaccinations. Consult your doctor before undergoing vaccination.

◆ Some DMARDs may cause birth defects. When applicable, this is pointed out under the heading: "Women of Childbearing Age." For more information, see Table 10-1. As indicated, the cytotoxic drugs may affect spermatogenesis (sperm formation). In the case of relevant drugs, the heading reads "Women of Childbearing Age/Men." Men who intend to father a child should discuss the matter with their physician.

MORE ABOUT INDIVIDUAL DMARDS

Cytotoxic Agents

Rheumatologists inherited the cytotoxic agents from cancer therapy. Don't be alarmed. The dose used for the treatment of arthritis is negligible when compared to the doses used in cancer therapy. The word *cytotoxic* means "cell poison." Indeed, cytotoxic agents affect a cell's DNA (genetic blueprint). This in turn reduces cell proliferation. The agents most markedly affect the rapidly dividing cells of the immune system, the hair follicles, and those lining the gastrointestinal tract.

Cytotoxic agents target cell division of the more rapidly dividing cells. Regular monitoring, especially during the initial phase of therapy, alerts the physician to potentially serious side effects.

Since cytotoxic agents interfere with DNA, they may cause birth defects. Sexually active patients, therefore, must use effective methods of birth control. Both men and women must discontinue medication in a timely fashion before undertaking pregnancy/impregnation. Because many of these drugs also enter breast milk, breastfeeding must be discussed with the physician.

Azathioprine (Imuran)

This anticancer agent was the first drug of this type approved by the Food and Drug Administration (FDA) for use in RA. Currently, it is mostly used in combination therapy.

How does azathioprine work? The drug interferes with the proliferation of lymphocytes.

Onset: 6 to 8 weeks.

Effectiveness: Moderate.

Side effects: Serious. Lowered white cell count, blood abnormalities (as manifested by increased bleeding and bruising), liver toxicity (as manifested by nausea, vomiting, jaundice, clay-colored stools), increased rate of infection. Slightly increased cancer risk. Hair loss, rashes, nausea, vomiting, diarrhea.

Precautions: Avoid contact with people with active infections. Contact your physician if you:

◆ Develop a fever, sore throat, or cough

◆ Note bleeding or easy bruising

◆ Develop jaundice

◆ Have changes in urine or stool color

Special tests: Close monitoring of liver function and blood counts.

Women of childbearing age/men: Discontinue at least 30 days (including one menstrual cycle) before trying to become pregnant. Azathioprine enters breast milk. Many physicians now permit the drug to be taken during pregnancy because it does not seem to cause birth defects or otherwise affect the fetus.

Dosage: 50–200 mg/day. To reduce gastrointestinal (GI) irritation, take medication with meals.

Cyclophosphamide (Cytoxan)

Cyclophosphamide is a powerful agent with serious side effects. It can be lifesaving for patients suffering from aggressive RA.

How does cyclophosphamide work? The drug promotes cell death, thereby decreasing the number of circulating B and T lymphocytes.

Onset: 2 weeks to 3 months

Effectiveness: Highly effective.

Side effects: Depressed red and white blood cells, reversible hair loss, sharply increased susceptibility to infection, nausea. Oral administration may cause bladder irritation, sometimes causing urinary blood loss. While on cyclophosphamide, drink large amounts of fluids, which "wash" the bladder.

Using the lowest possible dose and/or administering the drug for short periods of time minimizes serious side effects.

Long-term usage of cyclophosphamide in patients with urinary abnormalities may result in bladder cancer. There is also a slight, delayed (10 years) increase in the incidence of other types of cancer.

Precautions: Contact your physician if you experience any of the following:

- Any unusual symptoms
- Body temperature above 100°F (38°C)
- Stomach pain
- Rash, sore throat, or cough
- Sudden, severe, or unusual headache
- Painful and/or frequent urination
- Blood in urine

Special tests: Close monitoring of urine and bladder function, and frequent blood counts.

Women of childbearing age/men: Menstruation may cease when high doses of cyclophosphamide are used for long periods of time. Cyclophosphamide may cause sterility in both men and women. Birth-control pills may mitigate this effect. As a precautionary measure, patients may bank sperm or embryos but not eggs. Cyclophosphamide can cause birth defects and must be discontinued at least 30 days and one menstrual cycle before attempting pregnancy. The drug enters breast milk and breastfeeding is contraindicated.

Dosage: Variable. Cyclophosphamide can be taken as a pill or by intravenous injection. Side effects (hair loss, sterility, bladder toxicity) are decreased when the drug is given intermittently (*pulse* or *bolus* administration) at high dosage. Such a schedule does not reduce the effectiveness of the medication. The most common dosage schedule of cyclophosphamide pulse treatment is monthly for 6 months, then every 3 months for another year.

Cyclosporine (Neoral, Sandimmune)

Cyclosporine, a drug that made organ transplantation a realistic medical option, is used in patients with severe, active RA who have not responded to, or were intolerant of, one or more major DMARDs, including methotrexate, gold, and penicillamine. Cyclosporine is sometimes used in combination with methotrexate.

How does cyclosporine work? The drug is a powerful immunosuppressant.

Onset: Weeks to months.

Effectiveness: Highly effective.

Side effects: Because cyclosporine can cause severe liver and kidney toxicity, it is contraindicated in people with preexisting liver or kidney damage. Nausea, vomiting, diarrhea. Bleeding, tender or swollen gums, fluid retention, loss of appetite, high blood pressure, tremors.

Precautions: Cyclosporine increases the susceptibility to infection. Discuss vaccination with your physician.

Special tests: Kidney function must be monitored closely during therapy. Blood tests to determine concentration of drug in blood. Complete assessment of liver function.

Women of childbearing age/men: Cyclosporine may cause missed menstrual periods, as well as infertility in both men and women. Cyclosporine may cause birth defects and must be discontinued 1 to 3 months before considering pregnancy.

Dosage: Pills, suspension; 200–400 mg/day as a single or divided dose. Take at the same time each day, with or in between meals.

Leflunomide (Arava)

Leflunomide was approved for the treatment of RA in September 1998. It is one of the few drugs specifically developed for the treatment of RA.

How does leflunomide work? The drug apparently interferes with the proliferation of lymphocytes, especially T cells. This in turn reduces joint destruction.

Onset: Improvement evident after 1 month and stabilized after 3 to 6 months.

Effectiveness: Overall effectiveness is not known, but in some clinical trials the drug was more effective than methotrexate.

Side effects: The drug may affect liver and kidney function. Most commonly, patients develop diarrhea, headache, respiratory infection, weight loss, and temporary hair loss. The drug does not seem to increase the incidence of cancer.

Precautions: The FDA issued a strong warning about liver toxicity.

Special tests: Initially, monthly liver function tests. Elevated liver enzymes may return to normal with decreased dosage.

Women of childbearing age/men: The drug may cause birth defects and should not be used by pregnant women, as well as men or women contemplating pregnancy/impregnation. Since leflunomide has an extremely long half-life (it takes the body a long time to get rid of the drug), patients should undergo an 11-day elimination course with cholestyramine (8 g/3 times/day) before initiating pregnancy/fertilization. After the elimination procedure, blood should be checked for presence of the drug. Without the drug elimination procedure, some leflunomide might remain in the body for up to 2 years.

Dosage: Treatment with leflunomide is initiated with a loading dose of 100 mg/day for 3 days, thereafter 20 mg/day.

Methotrexate

Methotrexate is currently the most commonly and successfully used DMARD for the treatment of RA. Occasionally, people worry that methotrexate was inherited from cancer therapy. Let us stress that RA and cancer are unrelated. Besides, the dosages of methotrexate used for the treatment of RA are much lower than those used in cancer therapy. Taking methotrexate does not increase a person's risk of developing cancer.

How does methotrexate work? Methotrexate interferes with the cell's access to folic acid, an essential nutrient. This type of drug is therefore called an antimetabolite (disrupting the normal life cycle of the cell). Antimetabolites affect the growth of abnormal cells much more than they affect the growth of normal cells.

Onset: Within 4 weeks.

Effectiveness: Approximately 60 percent of patients suffering from RA respond to methotrexate, some experiencing complete remission of symptoms. The rapid improvement noted after methotrexate therapy suggests that the drug has some anti-inflammatory properties.

Side effects: At the dosages used for the treatment of RA, the drug is fairly well tolerated. Nevertheless, patients should be closely monitored to prevent serious side effects. The most common side effects are GI upset including nausea, vomiting, loss of appetite, diarrhea, and mouth sores. Most of these subside with continuous usage.

A rare but serious side effect is a peculiar type of lung inflammation beginning with a dry cough, which requires immediate cessation of therapy. The condition occurs mostly in smokers.

Other rare side effects include liver damage, as well as a slight increase in the incidence of cancer of the lymph nodes.

Precautions: Methotrexate interferes with many other drugs, including antibiotics, especially Bactrim, Septra, and Cotrim. Call your doctor if you develop a fever or the flu. Do not consume any alcohol while on methotrexate.

Special tests: Close monitoring of liver function to identify possible cirrhosis (inflammation of the liver); blood counts to detect leukopenia (low white blood cells) and damage to the bone marrow.

Women of childbearing age/men: Methotrexate may interfere with menstruation (cessation or irregularities), but does not affect fertility. The drug can cause abortions and birth defects and must be discontinued at least 30 days, including one menstrual cycle, before attempting pregnancy. Methotrexate passes into breast milk and breastfeeding is contraindicated.

Methotrexate may lower sperm count, but the effect is reversible. It is not known whether birth defects can be caused by men taking methotrexate, and it is recommended that the drug be discontinued 3 months prior to attempting impregnation.

Dosage: Methotrexate is most effective when the entire dose is taken once a week. This allows the body to recover between doses. On the dosage day, the entire dose may be taken at once, or split into two or three portions during the morning, noon, and night within a period of 12 hours.

Methotrexate is either taken by mouth (pills or liquid) or by injection. The usual starting dose is 7.5 mg once a week. Over time, the dosage may be increased to 20 mg once a week. Folic acid supplementation (1 mg/day) is indicated.

Immunomodulators

Etanercept (Enbrel)

Etanercept is the first in a new class of RA drugs known as biological response modifiers. Etanercept's long-term effects are unknown. The drug, however, offers hope for patients who do not respond to traditional DMARDs. Unfortunately, Etanercept is very expensive and reimbursement by major insurance companies must be negotiated on a case-by-case basis. The following information is derived from short-term usage.

How does etanercept work? The tumor necrosis factor (TNF) is one of the cytokines responsible for the amplification of the abnormal immune response and inflammatory processes characteristic of RA (see Chapter 5). Etanercept competes as a TNF receptor, which ties up TNF before it reaches the surface of the cell. This decreases the acute self-perpetuating inflammation.

Onset: Usually 1 to 2 weeks, maximum effect after 3 months.

Effectiveness: The drug is quite effective in 60–70 percent of patients. It has the potential to stop and/or prevent joint erosion and to markedly improve the clinical state of patients.

Side effects: Injection site reactions (37 percent), but they do not require discontinuation of the drug. Slightly increased rate of minor upper respiratory infections, sinusitis, and a few more serious infections.

Precautions: Preexisting infections may cause death.

Women of childbearing age: In animal studies, etanercept did not harm fetuses.

Dosage: 25 mg subcutaneously, twice a week at an interval of 72–96 hours. The drug does not interfere with methotrexate, corticosteroids, salicylates, and NSAIDs. It is self-injected under the skin. The manufacturer provides all the necessary equipment (drug powder, solvent, syringe, etc.) and clear instructions for administration.

Remicade (Infliximab)

Like entanercept, this drug is a TNF-alpha inhibitor. Currently, the drug is approved for the treatment of active Crohn's disease and RA. Its long-term effects are unknown.

How does remicade work? See etanercept, though there are slight differences in the mechanism of action of these agents.

Onset: Rapid, within weeks.

Effectiveness: 60–70 percent of patients.

Side effects: Fever, low blood pressure, fatigue, infections, primarily in patients with skin ulcers or skin infections. Very rarely, Remicade can cause lupus.

Precautions: Preexisting infections.

Women of childbearing age: See etanercept.

Dosage: 3 mg/kg given as a single IV infusion.

Miscellaneous Agents: Gold (Aurothioglucose, Gold Thioglucose, Solganal), Gold sodium thiomalate (Myochrysine), and Auranofin (Ridaura)

First used in 1929, gold salts are the oldest DMARD in continuous use. Until 1985, the drug had to be injected. Today, an oral preparation is available.

How does gold work? Even after all this time, it is not exactly known how gold works. The compounds have antimicrobial effects and seem to suppress some of the white blood cells (B and T lymphocytes and polymorphonuclear lymphocytes) that promote inflammation (see Chapter 5.)

Onset: Gradual amelioration of symptoms over a period of 6 months.

Effectiveness: Toxic reactions force discontinuation in 25 to 50 percent of patients. Of those who continue, 20 percent experience complete remission and 60 to 70 percent are markedly improved.

Side effects: Skin rash, mouth ulcers, kidney damage as manifested by proteinuria (protein in urine), stomach upset, increased sensitivity to sunlight, metallic taste, sore, swollen, and/or bleeding gums.

Oral gold is less toxic than when injected. Diarrhea, which may abate, occurs in 40 percent of patients. Patients must report any toxic reaction (skin rashes, stomach upsets) promptly to their physician.

Precautions: Cannot be used in patients allergic to test dose.

Special tests: Thorough medical examination, blood counts, and complete laboratory tests, especially during initiation of therapy.

Women of childbearing age: The drug used to be discontinued at least 30 days, including one menstrual cycle before attempting pregnancy, but today gold therapy may only be discontinued during part of the pregnancy or not at all. Discuss with your physician. Breastfeeding is contraindicated.

Dosage: Intramuscular gold: After a test dose of 10 mg, 25 mg are given 1 week later, thereafter 50 mg/week. Patients usually respond to therapy after having received 300–700 mg total. After maximum improvement has been achieved, dosage is decreased to 50 mg once every 2 weeks for 1–2 months, then to 50 mg once a month.

Oral gold: One 3 mg capsule twice a day.

Antimalarials

Hydroxychloroquine and Chloroquine

Like aspirin, the antimalarial drugs were first obtained from the bark of a tree, this one growing in Peru. Folk medicine had it that the bark of the cinchona tree contained a drug that cured malaria. In 1820, two scientists isolated quinine, and it was commonly used for the treatment of malaria. Seventy years later, it was used for the first time for the treatment of some rheumatic disorders.

Quinine itself is rather toxic. Some of its derivatives are more easily tolerated. The two that concern us here are hydrochloroquine and chloroquine. Since the 1950s, both have been extensively used for the treatment of RA.

How do the antimalarials work? The antimalarials are powerful anti-inflammatory and immunosuppressive agents with marked antimicrobial activity. The drugs inhibit the lysosomal enzymes, decrease the activity of the lymphocytes and PMNs, and reduce the release of interleukin 1.

Onset: Their onset of action is slow. Maximal antirheumatic effectiveness is only achieved after 6 months.

Effectiveness: Several long-term studies have shown the drugs to be effective in 60 to 70 percent of patients, with some experiencing complete remission and others experiencing marked improvement.

A comparison of the relative value of hydroxychloroquine and chloroquine was inconclusive, but since hydroxychloroquine has fewer side effects, it is the antimalarial of choice.

Side effects: The most potentially serious side effect is damage to the retina of the eye. Other side effects include allergy to the drug, gastrointestinal disturbances (heartburn, nausea, vomiting), rashes, and minor neurologic manifestations (headaches, insomnia, nervousness). All side effects are mild and transient, and the antimalarials are usually well tolerated.

Precautions: Should not be used in the presence of psoriasis, porphyria, or concomitantly with gold.

Special tests: A baseline eye examination (slit-lamp examination, visual fields, acuity, other) precedes the initiation of the drug. Repeat ocular examinations are scheduled every 6 months.

Women of childbearing age: The use of hydroxychloroquine during pregnancy is being reevaluated. Many physicians argue for its continued use during pregnancy, particularly in patients suffering from systemic lupus.

Dosage: Usually 200–600 mg/day in one or two doses.

Minocycline (Minocin, Dynacin)

Minocycline is an antibiotic belonging to the tetracycline family.

How does minocycline work? The drug is an antimicrobial agent, but its mode of action in RA is unknown.

Onset: The onset of action of the drug is slow (months).

Effectiveness: Not yet known

Side effects: Usually well tolerated. Gastrointestinal disturbances, skin rashes, vaginal infections, dizziness, and headaches occur occasionally.

Precautions: People sensitive to tetracycline antibiotics should not use the drug. The drug should be used cautiously in patients with impaired kidney function. The drug decreases prothrombin time, and patients on anticoagulant therapy may require a dosage adjustment.

Women of childbearing age: Discontinue the drug months before initiating pregnancy.

Dosage: 200 mg/day in divided dosage.

Penicillamine (Cuprimine)

Penicillamine, a waste product of penicillin, binds heavy metals such as copper and iron. It is moderately effective in the treatment of RA except in patients with marked extra-articular features such as rheumatoid vasculitis (inflammation of the veins and arteries). Penicillamine is rarely used today because of its severe side effects.

How does penicillamine work? It is presumed that penicillamine decreases the activity of the T lymphocytes and inhibits the release of the lysosomal enzymes that promote cartilage destruction.

Onset: Up to 12 weeks.

Effectiveness: In approximately 50 percent of patients.

Side effects: Itching and skin rashes, stomach upset, alteration of taste (usually disappears after 2 to 3 months of usage), decreased blood counts.

Precautions: Use with caution in people allergic to penicillin. Penicillamine is contraindicated in the presence of kidney disease, and for patients receiving gold, cytotoxic (immunosuppressive) DMARDs, or phenylbutazone.

Special tests: Complete blood counts, platelets, and urine analysis every 2 weeks during initial 6 months, and monthly thereafter.

Women of childbearing age: Discontinue drug months before initiating pregnancy.

Dosage: Initially, 250 mg/day for 2–3 months, then increased to 375–500 mg/day. If response is insufficient, increase to a maximum of 750 mg/day after another 2–3 months.

Sulfasalazine (Azulfidine)

Dr. Nanna Svartz, a Swedish rheumatologist, believed that a still unidentified infectious agent caused RA. In 1939, she combined sulfonamide, an effective antimicrobial drug, with salicylic acid, forming sulfasalazine. Dr. Svartz used the drug, at the time the only one ever to be specifically used for the treatment of RA, successfully for a number of patients.

Other physicians used sulfasalazine, but concluded that gold salts were a better drug, and sulfasalazine fell into disuse. In the meantime, sulfasalazine turned out to be a lifesaving treatment for recurrent ulcerative colitis.

All that was half a century ago. During the past decade, there has been renewed interest in the use of sulfasalazine for the treatment of RA. Today, it is mostly used in combination with other DMARDs.

How does sulfasalazine work? It appears to reduce joint inflammation by inhibiting the migration of white blood cells, especially PMN migration, to reduce lymphocyte response, and to reduce the development of blood vessels supplying inflamed joint tissue.

Onset: 4 weeks to 3 months.

Effectiveness: As effective as gold and penicillamine.

Side effects: The drug usually is well tolerated. Side effects include gastrointestinal discomfort, loss of appetite, nausea, vomiting, and headaches. Less commonly, the drug causes skin rashes, fever, tinnitus (ringing in the ears), and orange-yellow discoloration of urine and skin. Side effects decrease with usage.

Precautions: Sulfasalazine should not be taken by people allergic to sulfa drugs. The drug should be used cautiously by those suffering from bronchial asthma or severe allergies. Drink plenty of water while taking sulfasalazine.

Women of childbearing age/men: It is not known whether sulfasalazine affects the human fetus. Unless absolutely necessary, it is advisable to discontinue the drug 30 days, including one menstrual cycle, before attempting pregnancy. Traces of sulfasalazine appear in breast milk, and breastfeeding is contraindicated. Sulfasalazine can cause reversible infertility in men.

Dosage: Initially, 1 g/day in two to four divided doses. Dosage is increased to 2–3 g/day in two to four divided doses over a period of 3–4 months. Take medication after meals. Enteric-coated tablets that reduce stomach upset are available.

◆ CHAPTER ◆

9

Corticosteroids

<hr>

The chapter explores the discovery of the corticosteroids and reviews the role they play in RA. Emphasis is placed on taking these powerful medications safely.

THE DISCOVERY OF THE CORTICOSTEROIDS

In July 1948, a young woman was admitted to the Mayo Clinic in Rochester, Minnesota, one of the foremost medical centers in the United States. Janet W. (not her real name) was 29 years old, but looked 50. Her body was ravaged by 5 years of unremitting RA. Her joints were stiff, swollen, and extremely tender. Her right hip was almost completely destroyed and she could barely shuffle along the hospital's corridor. Janet was in constant pain.

Dr. Philip S. Hench, chief of rheumatology, tried all available treatments—injections of gold salts, hot baths, massive doses of vitamin E, extended time in the sun—all to no avail. He was about to give up when he remembered a hormone-like substance, compound E, prepared during World War II in Rahway, New Jersey, by Merck.

During the 1940s, medical attention centered on the hormones, the messengers of the body emitted by ductless glands such as the thyroid. A mere 25 years earlier, two Canadian scientists had discovered that insulin, made by the islet cells embedded in the pancreas, saved the life of previously doomed diabetics. Other miracles followed. Hundreds of different hormones regulate the body's key functions including blood pressure, sexual function, digestion, pregnancy, and sleep. The body produces hormones in minute amounts. Pharmaceutical companies were hard put to produce them in quantities large enough to be used as medications.

At the time, scientists also investigated the dozens of hormones made by the almond-sized adrenal glands, whose malfunction caused disease and even death. Scientists knew that the adrenals consist of an inner medulla (center) and outer cortex (shell or rind), and that both of these produce various hormones. Eventually, a German-born chemist, Tadeus Reichstein, managed to extract 25 of the hormones produced by the adrenal cortex. This substance had the same overall structure as cholesterol and the sex hormones.

World War II was raging and a rumor circulated that German scientists had discovered a specific hormone manufactured by the adrenal cortex and were administering it to the pilots of the Luftwaffe to help them overcome the stress of high altitude and long flights. Before this information was proven false, scientists at Merck pharmaceuticals undertook the very difficult task of preparing adrenal hormones. The preparation that concerns us was called compound E. It had been very difficult to prepare, and, all in all, Merck had 5 grams of compound E. By 1948, nobody had found a use for it, but fortunately one of the scientists who had assisted in the manufacture of compound E was Dr. Edward C. Kendall, who, like Hench, now worked at the Mayo Clinic.

When Dr. Hench saw the plight of his patient, he decided to act on an old hunch. In 1929, Hench had noticed that longstanding RA often remitted in patients who suffered from jaundice, were pregnant, or underwent surgery. The common denominator of these three conditions seemed to be stress. Hench believed that when stressed, the body produced an antirheumatic factor, which he called compound X. The fact that compound E was believed to alleviate stress suggested that it might be his "imagined" compound X. Hench discussed the matter with his friend and colleague, Edward Kendall, and this is how Merck's last gram of compound E arrived in Rochester, Minnesota.

Hench received the drug on September 21, 1948, and promptly injected Janet W. with it. That day and the next, Janet's RA continued unabated, but on day 3, Janet woke up without pain. The swelling in her joints subsided and she could walk. Four days later, after only seven daily doses, she was able to go out shopping. A miracle!

By then, her doctor had almost run out of compound E, or cortisone, as it was called from then on. Hench made a desperate call to Merck. No, they did not have any more cortisone, but they promised to marshal their forces. Within days, the pharmaceutical manufacturer sent another gram of cortisone to Hench. Eventually, Hench had enough cortisone to try it on 14 other severely impaired patients suffering from RA. Cortisone relieved these patients of their symptoms.

Philip Hench was a cautious doctor. During his career, he had seen too many arthritis "cures." Any day, he expected his patients to relapse, but after weeks and months, they were still symptom-free. In April 1949, Dr. Hench shared his news with his colleagues at a scientific meeting in Atlantic City. Hench showed a film of RA patients painfully tottering and shuffling along the corridors of the Mayo Clinic. After they received the cortisone injections, these same patients climbed steps, smiled, and even danced. Before the film was over, the audience gave Hench a standing ovation. The following year, the Nobel prize committee in Sweden awarded Edward C. Kendall, Philip S. Hench, and Tadeus Reichstein a Nobel prize.

Even at the triumphant meeting, Dr. Hench stressed that cortisone was not a permanent remedy. He knew that the drug had to be administered regularly. "The hormone is not a cure," he kept repeating. "Cortisone is the fireman who puts out the fire; it is not the carpenter who rebuilds the damaged house."

From the beginning, Hench was aware that cortisone increases blood sugar levels, and depletes the body of certain minerals including potassium and calcium. He knew that the agent could cause fatigue, muscle weakness, stomach ulcers, cataracts, impaired wound healing, moon facies (deposits of fat in the face that make it look swollen), and other severe side effects. Early on, however, awareness of these side effects seemed less important than the fact that cortisone was able to subjugate crippling arthritis. The newspapers touted the news and arthritis patients from all over America clamored for cortisone.

At first, the drug was unavailable. Each one of Hench's injections had cost Merck $1,000 in 1948. Eventually, however, Merck and other drug companies were able to mass produce cortisone and other closely related chemical substances. Today, corticosteroids (prednisone, betamethasone, dexamethasone, hydrocortisone) are widely used in medicine. Their use is crucial for patients suffering from respiratory diseases such as asthma, severe gastrointestinal diseases such as ulcerative colitis, and many rheumatic disorders. They are extremely powerful agents and must be used with caution. Hench's contribution to rheumatology must never be forgotten.

MODE OF ACTION

Ironically, Hench's idea of the beneficial hormone-like effect of the corticosteroids was all wrong. The drugs work because they are powerful anti-inflammatory agents. Like the NSAIDs, corticosteroids interrupt the prostaglandin cascade, but more efficiently. At high doses the steroids are immunosuppressive.

Since their discovery, the use of corticosteroids in rheumatology has waxed and waned. At first they were widely used. Then physicians and patients became terribly scared of their powerful side effects. Today, physicians use these powerful agents with more expertise, most often in conjunction with one or more of the DMARDs discussed in Chapter 8.

USE OF CORTICOSTEROIDS

Currently, corticosteroids are commonly used in the treatment of several rheumatic diseases, including RA. The drugs can be taken orally or by injection. Sometimes, especially for patients suffering from osteoarthritis (OA), corticosteroids are injected directly into the joint. Your physician will try very hard to use these drugs for short periods of time only and at the lowest possible dose. Many patients are able to tolerate low dosages of these drugs for years without significant side effects. Table 9–1 lists commonly prescribed corticosteroid preparations. In addition to the proprietary products listed, many generic products are available.

TABLE 9-1. Commonly Prescribed Corticosteroids

Cortisone acetate (compound E) (Cortone Acetate)

Dexamethasone (Decadron)

Fludrocortisone acetate (Florinef Acetate)

Hydrocortisone (Cortef, Hydrocortone)

Methylprednisolone (Medrol)

Prednisolone (Prelone)

Prednisone (Deltasone)

Triamcinolone (Aristocort)

DOSAGE

The side effects to any drug are usually dose related—that is, the higher the dose, the greater the risk of side effects. The dosage of corticosteroids (in terms of prednisone) is subdivided as follows by the American College of Rheumatology (ACR).

Low Dose: Up to 7.5 mg/day

There is a low risk of side effects with this dose. This amount almost corresponds to levels naturally present in the body and is well tolerated during prolonged use. (The body normally produces the equivalent of 7.5 mg prednisone a day, mostly in the late afternoon.) At this low dosage, side effects are generally acceptable. There may, however, be bone loss. The administration of corticosteroids as a drug shuts down the body's mechanism for making its own hormone. Even low-dose corticosteroids must be discontinued gradually in order to give the body a chance to restart making its own.

Intermediate Dose: 7.5 to 20 mg/day

Intermediate dosage is well tolerated when used for 1 month or less. In patients with active disease, the benefits of prolonged use may outweigh the potential side effects.

High Dose: 20 to 60 mg/day

High-dose corticosteroids may be recommended in case of severe systemic disease. Dosage should be reduced whenever possible.

Extremely High Dose: 100 to 1,000 mg/day

Extremely high dosage is used only in exceptional cases for short periods of time.

MEDIC ALERT SYSTEM BRACELETS

Long-term corticosteroid usage affects the body's metabolism (see "Side Effects"). Be sure to wear a Medic Alert System bracelet so that the medication can be administered properly during medical emergencies (e.g., surgery, accidents).

SIDE EFFECTS

The hormones produced by the adrenal glands and their synthetic counterparts control many important body functions including the regulation of blood sugar, fat, salt and water metabolism, and growth. The hormones participate in the regulation of immune function. These essential functions are altered when corticosteroids are given in therapeutic doses.

Corticosteroid therapy profoundly impacts on carbohydrate, protein, and fat metabolism, as well as water and electrolyte balance. The drugs must be taken especially cautiously by patients for whom diabetes, high blood pressure, or ulcers are a concern. As always, it is important to be familiar with the side effects of any drug you take so that you can discuss them with your physician. Table 9–2 reviews the side effects encountered during corticosteroid therapy. This classification into very common, common, occasional, and less common side effects is derived from the Arthritis Foundation booklet "Corticosteroids."

TABLE 9-2. Side Effects Commonly Encountered During Corticosteroid Therapy

- *Very common side effects:* Weight gain (see this chapter and Chapter 11), increased appetite, and insomnia. Corticosteroids promote weight gain because they enhance both fluid retention and body fat storage. Promptly report swelling of the legs to your physician. Corticosteroids seem to affect the nervous system. Some patients feel anxious, others buoyant, others depressed. Corticosteroids affect sleep (see Chapter 14), so it is helpful to take these drugs early in the day.

- *Common side effects:* Alteration of body fat distribution. Corticosteroids promote the deposition of fat in facial tissue (moon face), abdominal and shoulder regions. Heartburn and stomach ulcers are aggravated by concomitant use of NSAIDs. Altered hair growth (thinning and/or excessive growth). Wasting of muscle tissue, mild muscle weakness, especially in arms or legs, blurred vision, cataracts, easy bruising of the skin. Delayed wound healing, acne, suppression of menstrual cycle, osteoporosis (see text), red or purple stretch marks. Osteonecrosis, or bone death, characterized by abrupt onset of severe pain. The condition is caused by inadequate blood supply to the affected area. Early stages of osteonecrosis are treated conservatively (analgesics, maintenance of muscle strength, stress reduction of affected area by means of assistive devices). Later stages may require surgery.

- *Occasional side effects:* High blood pressure, elevated blood sugar.

- *Less common side effects:* Glaucoma, severe muscle weakness, psychosis, serious infections due to suppression of the immune system.

Weight Gain

One of the most unpleasant side effects of corticosteroids is that they profoundly affect the manner in which the body handles food, thereby causing a characteristic weight gain. Fat tissue is deposited around the face (moon facies), on the back (dowager's hump), and around the center of the abdomen. Often, the drugs also cause ravenous hunger.

Eugenia Zuckerman, the world-famous flutist, had to take high doses of corticosteroids for a number of months. Afterward, she and her sister, Julie R. Ingelfinger, M.D., wrote a book entitled *Coping with Prednisone* (St. Martin's Press, 1997) that should prove most helpful to anyone taking these powerful medications for a long time. Chapter 11 relates Zuckerman's experiences and suggests ways of eating healthily while on corticosteroids.

Mood Swings

People on high-dose corticosteroids describe themselves as vulnerable, swinging from exhilaration and ecstasy to the deepest sorrow. The confident feel panicky, the laid-back become overanxious, the cautious feel reckless, the silent feel talkative, and the trusting become suspicious. There is no pattern to these mood changes except that the emotional response to cortisosteroid therapy is highly variable. Some patients remain unaffected, but most patients report being "off balance."

When to Call the Doctor

If you are taking corticosteroids, call your doctor if you notice the following:

◆ Any unusual symptom

◆ Temperature above 100°F (38°C)

◆ Stomach pain, vomiting, gastrointestinal bleeding, or black stools

◆ Increased thirst or increased urination

◆ Sudden, severe, or unusual headache

◆ Significant change in mood or thinking

TAPERING CORTICOSTEROIDS

Corticosteroids represent a "high" to which the body adjusts very quickly. When withdrawn, your body may respond with muscle pain, nausea, weight loss, headaches, and even fever. Usually these symptoms are short-lived. Contact your physician if they persist, because withdrawal may have triggered a rheumatoid flare.

To avoid or minimize steroid withdrawal syndromes, corticosteroid medication is tapered (decreased gradually) over a period of weeks or even months. *Stopping steroids suddenly can be fatal.* Your doctor will prescribe your tapering regimen. It may involve a gradual decrease of daily dose, an alternate-day schedule (higher dose one day/lower dose the next), skipping alternate days, or adding a steroid-sparing drug such as Plaquenil, NSAIDs, or azathioprine to your regimen. To help your body get used to fewer or no corticosteroids, it is important that you adhere to the prescribed regimen.

CORTICOSTEROIDS AND OSTEOPOROSIS

Osteoporosis is a general risk factor for the world's rapidly aging, sedentary population. The risk is sharply increased by corticosteroid therapy. Bone, as explained in Chapter 3, is not inert but constantly replaces itself. Osteoblasts form new bone and osteoclasts dismantle bone. Bone mass is maximal in late adolescence or early adulthood. Hormonal changes starting at age 30 to 35 promote bone loss. Bones become thinner as people age. At first, bone loss is imperceptible, but after it exceeds a certain critical mass, the bones may fracture, and the person is said to suffer from osteoporosis.

Bone loss is a natural part of aging in both men and women. The condition occurs more often in women in part because they have a smaller skeleton and in part because bone needs estrogen to remain healthy. (Estrogen production declines at menopause.) In the United States alone, osteoporosis is estimated to affect 25 million women and is responsible for the hip fractures occurring in older people. Like arthritis, osteoporosis once seemed to be just another untreatable disease. This state of affairs has changed. Today, the risk of osteoporosis can be evaluated by a bone density scan, and treatment, including various combinations of estrogen replacement, alendronate (Fosamax), risedronate sodium (Actonel), etidronate (Didronel), thiazides, calcimar (Calcitonin), and exercise has become routine. These discoveries have had a major impact on the use of corticosteroids in RA.

Many of the mechanisms promoting osteoporosis have now been identified. Risk factors include:

◆ Decreased production of sex hormones

◆ Decreased absorption of calcium

- Insufficient calcium and vitamin D intake
- Lack of weight-bearing exercise
- Cigarette smoking
- Excessive use of alcohol or caffeine

A combination of drug therapy and risk factor reduction makes osteoporosis a preventable and treatable disease. These findings are extremely important for the 30 million Americans who are on corticosteroid therapy. Indeed, one of the most serious side effects of this often essential therapy is that these agents enhance many of the mechanisms promoting bone loss, particularly,

- Corticosteroids decrease the amount of calcium absorbed from food in the small intestine and increase the loss of calcium in the urine. Threatened by a decreased level of calcium in the blood, the body produces more parathyroid hormone, whose function is to mobilize calcium from bone. Corticosteroids stimulate osteoclasts (cells that break down bone) and inhibit osteoblasts (cells that build bone).
- Corticosteroids reduce sex hormone production—estrogen in women, testosterone in men. These hormones promote bone density.

In order to reduce the risk of osteoporosis, the ACR recommends the following lifestyle and possibly pharmacologic interventions for all patients on corticosteroid therapy:

- Maintain a calcium intake of 1,500 mg/day through diet and/or supplements.
- Maintain an adequate intake of vitamin D_3.
- If you smoke, stop.
- Limit or avoid alcohol consumption.
- Participate in weight-bearing exercises (30 to 60 minutes per day).

The prevention and treatment of osteoporosis is still in its infancy and therapies must be carefully monitored. The following modalities have been used successfully.

Hormone Replacement

- *Sex hormones:* Estrogen replacement therapy for postmenopausal women is advisable, unless contraindicated. Oral contraceptives may be effective in premenopausal women. Men with low testosterone levels may benefit from testosterone replacement.

♦ *Calcitonin:* This naturally occurring hormone participates in calcium metabolism. Its administration, by injection or intranasal spray, is effective in corticosteroid-induced osteoporosis.

Biphosphonates: Etidronate (Didronel), Alendronate (Fosamax), and Risedronate (Actonel)

These three bisphosphonates have proven effective in the prevention and treatment of osteoporosis including steroid-induced osteoporosis. It is recommended to take Fosamax and Actonel on an empty stomach with a full glass of water. Patients are cautioned to stand upright for at least 30 minutes until after breakfast. These maneuvers are meant to decrease esophageal irritation and improve absorption.

TIPS FOR TAKING CORTICOSTEROIDS

Corticosteroids are important drugs for the treatment of RA. With proper care, these drugs can be taken successfully during disease flares and even as part of your maintenance regimen. In summary:

♦ Be sure to take these agents as directed by your physician. Do not institute or discontinue them on your own. Increase and decrease corticosteroids as directed.

♦ Promptly report any side effects that you suspect are associated with the use of corticosteroids (blurred vision, sudden weight gain, swelling of legs, absence of menstruation, stomach upsets, excessive depression, undue nervousness).

♦ Follow your physician's recommendations for minimizing the side effects of the corticosteroids.

♦ Discuss stomach irritation with your physician. Consult Chapter 7 for ways to protect your stomach from irritation.

♦ Maintain a good diet with adequate intake of calcium and potassium. Avoid fattening foods and maintain adequate fluid intake. (For calcium intake, see Chapter 11.)

- Wear a Medic Alert System bracelet, because corticosteroids must be administered, even increased, during unusual stress (e.g., other disease, accidents, surgery).

- Be sure that all your health care providers are aware of the fact that you are taking corticosteroids.

- Since corticosteroids promote infection by decreasing the activity of your immune system, maintain strict hygiene. People on high-dose corticosteroid therapy should minimize direct contact with those having a contagious disease. You may even opt to discourage casual kissing.

- If possible, maintain your prescribed exercise regimen.

- Maintain joint protection even though your joints may hurt less.

◆ CHAPTER ◆

10

Pregnancy and RA

═══◊═══

This chapter discusses bearing a child when suffering from rheumatoid arthritis. The impact of medications on the unborn is reviewed in detail.

Since women of childbearing age are a primary target for developing RA, it goes without saying that a number of patients suffering from the disease want to bear children. Take heart. Most women with RA have given birth to normal, healthy infants. Labor and delivery are usually routine. A pregnancy, nevertheless, requires planning both from medical and lifestyle points of view. It's important to discuss your pregnancy with your physician, preferably before you actually become pregnant, so you and your doctor can develop an action plan.

Remember that RA is not inherited in the usual sense of the word. A predisposition to the disease may be passed on. Your baby will not suffer from rheumatoid arthritis.

MEDICAL ASPECTS

The decision to undertake a pregnancy most importantly hinges on the extent of your RA. The more severe the disease, the greater the physical disability, and the more drugs you must take to keep the disease in check. Few problems may be encountered by women with mild RA. Women with multiple joint involvement and aggressive disease may have a harder time both during the pregnancy and afterward.

Being pregnant seems to be good for many women with RA. During the first 3 months of the pregnancy, the disease abates in approximately 70 percent of patients. It was this remission that prompted Dr. Philip Hench of the Mayo Clinic to look for a biological factor (i.e., a body chemical) that protects women under these circumstances. This is how the physician discovered the corticosteroids, though these hormones were not the main factor in lessening RA during pregnancy.

MEDICATIONS

Most drugs cross the placenta and enter breast milk during lactation. Drugs that may harm the fetus are described as being *teratogenic*. Ideally, it is best to avoid taking any medication during pregnancy. This, however, is not always possible. Even though the RA may improve during pregnancy, it still has its ups and downs, and pregnant women may continue to require painkillers or short courses of corticosteroids. Fortunately, the unborn child is most sensitive to drugs soon after conception and during the early stages of the pregnancy, a time when the future mother can often do without medication.

The Food and Drug Administration (FDA), which evaluates the safety of drugs in the United States, has classified the DMARDs and other drugs commonly used for the treatment of RA with respect to their probable effects on the fetus. The classification of the FDA ranges from A to D and X, with A having no effect whatsoever on the fetus and D being relatively contraindicated; X is for unacceptable risk (see Table 10–1). Note that drugs such as methotrexate and cyclosporine, which affect cell development and are totally unacceptable and contraindicated during pregnancy, are not even listed in the table. Methotrexate, for example, must be stopped 3 months before conception to prevent birth defects. Any drug taken during pregnancy must be carefully examined and discussed with both your rheumatologist and your obstetrician. Both alcohol and cigarette smoke may have a deleterious effect on your baby. Consult Chapter 8 for more information on specific drugs.

TABLE 10-1. Possible Effect on Pregnancy of Selected Antirheumatic Drugs

Drug	FDA Risk Category*	Safety	Comments
Aspirin[†]	C/D[‡]	Variable, depends on dose and use	May cause maternal and fetal bleeding if administered near term; uncertain safety for high dose
Naproxen, ibuprofen, ketoprofen, and similar drugs[‡]	C/D[‡]	Variable, depends on dose and time of use	Experience largely accumulated through treatment of headache and dysmenorrhea; no major teratogenicity noted; use at term not advised.
Ketorolac[†]	C	Causes dystonia (muscle weakness) and neonatal death in animals	Insufficient human experience
Indomethacin[‡]	B/D[‡]	Variable, depends on dose and time of use	Rare cases of pulmonary hypertension if used at term
Prednisone	B	Generally safe	Small amount passes through the placenta, safe in lactation, but may suppress milk production
Methylprednisolone	B	Probably safe	Similar to prednisone, but fewer data available
Dexamethasone, betamethasone	C	Probably safe in late pregnancy	Major transport across placenta; used to induce fetal lung maturation
Hydroxychloroquine	Unclassified	Questionable safety	Small published experience indicates safety
Azathioprine	D	Safety uncertain	Large experience with renal transplant patients indicates no immediate danger to offspring if maternal dose is less than 2 mg/kg/day; rare reports of congenital anomalies, including immunodeficiency

Drug	FDA category	Risk	Comments
Cyclosporine	C	Probably safe	Little experience, none suggesting high fetal risk
Cyclophosphamide, methotrexate, chlorambucil	C§	Dangerous	Abortifacient (causes abortions), teratogenic
Leflunomide	X	Dangerous	Abortifacient (causes abortions), teratogenic, no data available
Heparin	B	Appears to be safe	Anticoagulant of choice; usually given subcutaneously twice daily; dose control essential for safety; causes osteoporosis
Low-molecular-weight heparin	B‖		
Warfarin	X	Teratogenic and possibly fetotoxic	Fetal warfarin syndrome when given in first trimester, may cause central nervous system (CNS) defects in second and third trimesters; risk of severe neonatal hemorrhage when given near term
Etanercept and Remicade	Unknown	Unknown	
Intravenous immunoglobulin	B‖	Unknown	Unknown

*Food and Drug Administration (FDA) pregnancy risk classification. A, controlled trials show no risk in humans; B, animal studies show no risk, *or* no definitive studies in humans; C, animal studies show risk, *or* no studies in humans, *or* no information; D, positive evidence of risk, risk:benefit ratio may be acceptable in some circumstances; X, fetal risk, risk:benefit ratio always unacceptable.

†All inhibitors of prostaglandin synthesis activity may inhibit labor and prolong gestation. There is also a risk of in utero closure of the ductus arteriosus (the connection in the circulation that allows the baby's blood flow to bypass the lungs).

‡Risk category D when used in the third trimester.

§Based on a critical need to use these drugs in cancer parents; X in RA category.

‖Assigned by Michael L. Lockshin, M.D.

Source: From Medical Disorders During Pregnancy, 3rd ed., by William M. Barron and Marshall D. Lindheimer. C. V. Mosby, St. Louis. Reproduced with permission.

POSTPREGNANCY FLARES

Unfortunately, even if RA goes into remission during pregnancy, most women flare during the first 8 weeks after delivery. The likelihood of this flare makes it important to suppress the disease just prior to and during delivery. Most physicians discontinue therapy during the early stages of the pregnancy and resume therapy late in the pregnancy, postpartum or postbreastfeeding. During pregnancy and breastfeeding, prednisone can be safely used to prevent flares.

A competent rheumatologist will be able to guide you through your pregnancy. He or she and your pediatrician can advise you on whether it is safe to breastfeed your baby.

NONMEDICAL CONSIDERATIONS

RA will not affect your actual pregnancy, and your pregnancy will not affect your RA. Pregnancy, nevertheless, will stress your body. To begin with, there is the added weight of the growing baby, which will impact on your joints. To evaluate this stress, the Arthritis Foundation suggests lifting and handling a 10-pound bag of potatoes. As always, rest will diminish the stress, and it is crucial that you rest as much as possible during your pregnancy. If you continue to work outside the house, try to lie down during your lunch hour.

The stress will increase after delivery. Babies require a tremendous amount of work. They tire out perfectly healthy mothers. Before undertaking a pregnancy, you should ask yourself whether you would be able to handle this extra stress. In contrast, not having a baby may be equally difficult. Making this decision will be extremely hard.

If you decide to have a baby, try to organize and coordinate a support system. The "Arthritis and Pregnancy" booklet published by the Arthritis Foundation provides many helpful tips. (You can obtain a copy by calling your local chapter.) These tips include matching the baby's paraphernalia to your specific needs. Some highlights are:

◆ Nursing or bottle-feeding the baby while sitting in a comfortable chair

◆ Using a high crib and bathinette so that you don't have to bend down while bathing or dressing your infant

◆ Using as many disposable items (diapers, bottles, etc.) as possible

◆ Using garments with Velcro fasteners

◆ Minimizing running around by having necessary implements close at hand

◆ Minimizing footwork by wearing an apron with deep pockets, in which to carry around small, frequently required necessities

The "Guide to Independent Living," published by the Arthritis Foundation, offers many sources for equipment (bathtubs, diapers, etc.) to help you care for your baby.

Make sure that you have plenty of help. Rest when you can. Exercise. Enjoy.

11

Nutrition and RA

————≈«(()»≈————

This chapter examines the interrelationship of nutrition and RA, provides simple tools for ensuring good nutrition, explores popular dietary supplements, provides lists of good food sources for calcium and micronutrients, and reviews the possible nutritional effects of medications used for the treatment of RA. Ways of eating healthily during corticosteroid therapy are suggested.

When you tell friends or colleagues that you have RA, chances are that someone will suggest a way of eating to improve your disease. Here are some examples:

"Stop eating red meat." *Or:*

"You mean to say that you eat tomatoes and other night-shade veg-etables?" *Or:*

"My uncle's mother-in-law's sister had a bad case of arthritis. Then she stopped drinking milk—or was it eating wheat?—and she was cured overnight." *Or:*

"Take honey and vinegar. You'll see that after a week or two you'll have less pain."

If you want to be technical, you'll notice that these recommendations include elimination diets and/or dietary supplements. Elimination diets involve avoidance of a particular food or food group, while supple-mentation involves adding specific foods.

Most of the recommendations made by your well-meaning friends fall into the category of "unproven remedies." It is not surprising that these crop up particularly often in connection with RA, whose course is so unpredictable and whose treatment may seem haphazard. Many unproven remedies are harmless. Some, however, result in inadequate nutrition, others are costly, and a few are dangerous. More importantly, the prolonged use of dietary therapy may delay seeking appropriate medical care. The belief that dietary changes will cure arthritis is so widespread that several scientists have investigated the subject in great detail.

FOOD AND RHEUMATOID ARTHRITIS

In a study of the food sensitivity of 704 patients suffering from RA, 28 percent reported that certain foods affected their arthritis. Ten percent reported a worsening, another 10 percent reported variable effects, and 5.5 percent improved when taking specific supplements, mostly vitamins and minerals (data from Tanner et al.: *Arthritis Care and Research,* December 1990).

A comparison of food intake and the prevalence of RA indicates that diet does not cause or cure RA. In rare cases, a person may be allergic to specific foods, and the allergy may produce rheumatic symptoms. Very occasionally, the inflammatory manifestations of RA may be aggravated by a specific combination of calories, protein, and fat. In general, a diet high in certain fats decreases inflammatory manifestations. Nutrition and specific nutritional supplements, nevertheless, play a crucial role in the management of RA. Some of these facts may be well known to you. Good nutrition is an important facet of maintaining good health, and in-depth knowledge of this important subject will help you.

THE COMPOSITION OF FOOD

Food consists of macronutrients, which the body needs in large amounts, and micronutrients, which are needed in only small amounts. Most foods, especially the prepared foods we eat, are mixtures of both macronutrients and micronutrients. A well-chosen food plan will supply the body with the nutrients it needs for good health.

Macronutrients

The macronutrients include proteins, carbohydrates, and fat. Each of these is put together from very simple units. During digestion in the gastrointestinal tract, the macronutrients are hydrolyzed (taken apart) into their components by enzymes. The resulting small units are absorbed from the gut into the blood and utilized.

Carbohydrates and Fats

Carbohydrates and fats are commonly called the energy nutrients because they supply the body with fuel. When energy supply exceeds demand (i.e., when you eat more calories than you need), the excess intake is stored as body fat. Conversely, when your body utilizes more energy than you take in, the body mobilizes its own tissues to meet the increased demand.

Carbohydrates are subdivided into simple carbohydrates and complex carbohydrates. Simple carbohydrates, such as table sugar, glucose, and fructose, consist of one or two building blocks; complex carbohydrates consist of hundreds of these same building blocks. Simple sugars taste sweet. They are naturally present in many foods (fruits, honey, milk) and are added in large amounts to cakes and other sweets. Simple sugars are quickly absorbed into the blood.

Dietary staple foods, such as rice and bread, consist of complex carbohydrates. The body converts complex carbohydrates into simple sugars in the gut. Complex carbohydrates release their sugar load slowly during digestion, thereby providing longer satiety and avoiding a "sugar high."

Fats

Fats are put together from fatty acids and glycerol. They can be saturated (lard, butter, others), monounsaturated (olive oil, others), or polyunsaturated (linolenic acid, others). For good health, the body requires some polyunsaturated fatty acids, and they are therefore referred to as essential fatty acids (EFAs).

Proteins

The word *protein* comes from the Greek and means "first." Indeed, protein—or rather the 21 different amino acids that make up the protein—is the essential building block of the body. The body utilizes these amino acids for growth, to replace worn parts and build enzymes, hormones, and other key substances that mastermind metabolism. (Metabolism is the sum total of the entire chemical processes that take place in an organism.) As essential as proteins are, the body needs only a small amount of them. Excess protein is burned for energy.

Micronutrients

Micronutrients include vitamins and minerals. Specific knowledge about their existence is more recent than information concerning the macronutrients. For centuries, however, scientists studied strange diseases that popped up under unusual circumstances. Sailors, for instance, might have developed scurvy during long sea voyages, if their diet lacked fresh fruit or vegetables. In certain parts of Indonesia, the native population developed beriberi—a neurological disease—when ordinary brown rice was replaced by the more elegant polished rice of the Dutch colonizers.

In time it was discovered that food contains small amounts of vitamins that are essential to life. Food also contains somewhat larger amounts of minerals whose regular consumption is also essential to good health.

Both vitamins and minerals have one or more specific jobs. By and large, vitamins play an important part in metabolism, and minerals are part of the body's structure. Calcium, for example, is part of bone, and iron is part of hemoglobin, the red coloring matter of blood.

Vitamins and minerals are absorbed from the gastrointestinal tract. Vitamins are subdivided into fat-soluble vitamins (vitamins A, D, E, and K) and water-soluble vitamins (vitamins B complex, C, and others).

Both vitamins and minerals are part of ordinary food. If they were not, our ancestors would have died out, since vitamin supplements are a recent development. Nevertheless, diets—old and new—may not be perfect, and we may profit from taking one multivitamin a day. Again, as in the case of protein, an excessive intake will not do any good. In the case of the fat-soluble vitamins, an excess can be harmful.

Even though vitamins are part of ordinary food, they require attention. Certain medications taken for the treatment of RA may interfere with vitamin absorption and/or utilization. In this case, there may be a need for supplementation (see "Medications and Food Intake for Patients with RA," later in this chapter).

HOW MUCH FOOD IS ENOUGH?

About 60 years ago, before World War II, the United States Army asked the United States Department of Agriculture (USDA) to determine whether the diet it fed its soldiers was healthy. The USDA determined the amount of proteins, vitamins, and minerals an individual should consume. This study resulted in the Recommended Daily Allowance—RDA—a person should eat. The RDA has been with us ever since. The USDA has now developed specific RDAs for 32 different population groups including infants, pregnant and lactating women, and older people. Remember that the RDA are not carved in stone. RDAs are simply helpful recommendations and should not interfere with your enjoyment of food. The complete RDA table is cumbersome. A shorter version is used to develop food labels that indicate the contribution of particular foods to your nutrition. The current U.S. RDA values are shown in Table 11–1.

The number of calories a person requires each day depends on age, body size, body weight, and physical activity. Most women require between 1,400 and 2,000 calories/day. Most men require between 1,600 and 2,400 calories/day. You may wish to discuss your particular requirements with a nutritionist.

TABLE 11-1. U.S. Recommended Dietary Allowances (U.S. RDA) for Adults and Children Over 4 Years of Age*

Protein†	65 g*	Vitamin B_6	2.0 mg
Protein, high quality	45 g*	Folacin	0.4 mg
Vitamin A	5,000 IU	Vitamin B_{12}	6 mcg
Vitamin C	50 mg	Phosphorus	1 g
Thiamin	1.5 mg	Iodine	150 mcg
Riboflavin	1.7 mg	Magnesium	400 mcg
Niacin	20 mg	Zinc	15 mg
Calcium	1 g	Copper	2 mg
Iron	18 mg	Biotin	0.3 mg
Vitamin D	400 IU	Pantothenic acid	10 mg
Vitamin E	30 IU		

*These U.S. RDAs are used by the food industry to develop food labels. When you look at a cereal box or can of tuna, you immediately see the daily percentage of a specific vitamin or protein that a serving size of that particular food will supply (see Table 11-2).
†The recommended intake of protein in the U.S. RDA depends on the quality of the protein.

FOOD LABELS

To help people eat a healthy diet, the food industry and the government decided to develop food labels that provide information about the nutrient content of the food in a manner that can be easily understood. In the RDA tables the requirement for nutrients is expressed in grams (g), milligrams (mg), micrograms (mcg), or International Units (IU). On food labels this same information is expressed in terms of percent (%). Put differently, the labels spell out the contribution that a particular food makes toward your daily nutrient requirement.

A whole can of tuna fish, for example, usually meets your daily protein requirement; a glass of milk only provides 30 percent of the calcium you require on a daily basis.

The food label also provides information on serving size (all nutrient information is provided in terms of serving size), calories, calories from fat, the type and amount of fat, sugar, and salt. A typical food label is shown in Table 11–2.

WHAT IS GOOD NUTRITION?

According to the latest research, a good diet consists of approximately:

◆   55 to 60 percent carbohydrates

◆   15 to 20 percent protein

◆   25 to 30 percent fat

Another device designed to help people eat a healthy diet is the food pyramid (Fig. 11–1). The base of the pyramid consists of staple foods (bread, cereal, rice, pasta) that are the backbone of diets throughout the world. The next level of the pyramid consists of fruits and vegetables that supply the bulk of the vitamins. The level above that consists of the protein foods, and the tip of the pyramid is for the fats, oils, and sweets that should be eaten sparingly. Table 11–3 provides good food sources for vitamins and minerals. Table 11–4 lists some good sources of calcium. For exact information, always read the food label.

TABLE 11-2. Information on a Typical Food Label

Toasted Oats		
Servings Per Container: 8		
Serving Size: 1 cup		
Amounts Per Serving	Dry	Cereal with 1/2 cup skim milk
Calories	120	160
Calories from Fat	15	20
		% Daily Values
Total Fat 2 g*		
Saturated Fat 0 g	0 %	3 %
Cholesterol	0 %	1 %
Sodium 210 mg	0 %	11 %
Potassium 65 mg	2 %	8 %
Total Carbohydrates 23 g	8 %	10 %
Dietary Fiber 2 g	8 %	8 %
Sugars 2 g		
Protein 3 g		
Vitamin A	25%	30 %
Vitamin C	25 %	25 %
Calcium	10 %	10 %
Iron	50 %	50 %
Vitamin D	10 %	25 %
Thiamine	25 %	30 %
Riboflavin	25 %	35 %
Niacin	25 %	25 %
Vitamin B$_6$	25 %	25 %
Folate	25 %	25 %

*Amount in Cereal
**Amount in Percent Daily Values as based on 2,000 calories/day diet.
Ingredients: Whole Oat Flour, Wheat Starch, Brown Sugar, Salt...
Ingredients: Vitamin C (Sodium Ascorbate, Ascorbic Acid,) Iron,
(Ferrous Fumerate) Vitamin A (Palmitate)...

Note: The cereal as well as the milk have been enriched so as to supply a greater percent of the RDA (daily values).

FIGURE 11-1. Food Pyramid

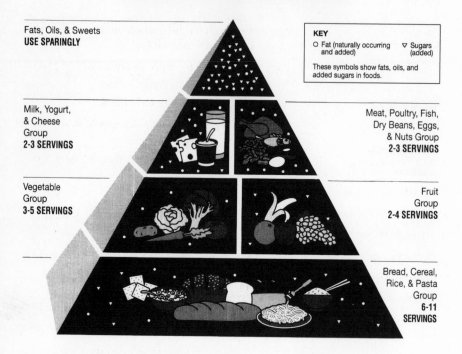

Food Guide Pyramid
A Guide to Daily Food Choices

Fats, Oils, & Sweets
USE SPARINGLY

KEY
○ Fat (naturally occurring   ▽ Sugars
   and added)   (added)

These symbols show fats, oils, and
added sugars in foods.

Milk, Yogurt,
& Cheese
Group
2-3 SERVINGS

Meat, Poultry, Fish,
Dry Beans, Eggs,
& Nuts Group
2-3 SERVINGS

Vegetable
Group
3-5 SERVINGS

Fruit
Group
2-4 SERVINGS

Bread, Cereal,
Rice, & Pasta
Group
**6-11
SERVINGS**

SERVING SIZE

The key to any good eating plan is learning to gauge the amount of food that corresponds to a serving size. Sometimes that is easy. Everybody knows what a medium-size apple means or a glass of milk. Gauging the size of a meat serving, french fries, or even bread is more difficult.

BODY WEIGHT

Weight plays a major role in the management of RA. Weight loss is an important aspect and often an initial symptom of active RA. Standard body weight tables may be misleading for people suffering from a chronic

TABLE II-3. Good Food Sources of Vitamins and Minerals

Vitamin A	Fortified dairy products, carrots and other orange and yellow vegetables, dark green and leafy vegetables
Vitamin B_1	Whole-grain and enriched cereals, pork, beef, peas, nuts, beans
Vitamin B_2	Milk, eggs, red meat, liver, fish, whole grains, enriched cereals, nuts, green leafy vegetables
Vitamin B_6	Meats, bananas, lima beans, eggs, peanuts, whole-grain cereals
Vitamin B_{12}	Milk, eggs, fish, seafood, fermented cheese
Folic acid	Liver, green leafy vegetables, potatoes, cereal products, fruit
Pantothenic acid	Peas, dried beans, lean meat, poultry, fish, whole-grain cereals
Niacin	Eggs, red meat, milk and dairy products
Biotin	Liver, cauliflower, salmon, carrots, bananas, soy flour, cereal, yeast
Vitamin C	Citrus fruit, peppers, broccoli, cabbage, tomatoes, potatoes
Vitamin D	Tuna, salmon, cod liver oil, vitamin D fortified milk
Vitamin E	Vegetable oil, whole-grain cereals, green leafy vegetables, wheat germ
Vitamin K	Green leafy vegetables, meats, dairy products
Calcium	Milk, egg, tuna, salmon, dairy products, tofu
Copper	Nuts, raisins, chocolate, mushrooms, kidneys
Iodine	Iodized salt, seafood
Iron	Red meat, egg yolks, liver, green vegetables (spinach, others), seafood, walnuts, beans
Magnesium	Broccoli, whole grain, enriched cereal products, meat
Phosphorus	Milk, fish, meat, whole grains, cottage cheese, yogurt, soft drinks

TABLE 11-4. Some Good Food Sources of Calcium

◆ Yogurt

◆ Milk including lactose-free and lactose-reduced milk

◆ Natural cheeses such as mozzarella, Cheddar, Swiss, and Parmesan

◆ Cottage cheese, ricotta cheese

◆ Soy-based beverages with added calcium

◆ Tofu, if made with calcium sulfate (read the ingredients list)

◆ Breakfast cereal with added calcium

◆ Canned fish with soft bones such as salmon and sardines (but high in salt)

◆ Fruit juice with added calcium

◆ Puddings made with milk

◆ Soup made with milk

◆ Dark green leafy vegetables such as collards and turnip greens

disease because they do not distinguish between muscle mass and body fat. If indicated, more accurate measurements can be obtained by using body mass index or triceps skinfold thickness measurements. Specific laboratory tests that measure serum protein, folic acid, or vitamin blood levels may be ordered by physicians who suspect that their patients suffer from protein calorie malnutrition.

Patients experiencing weight loss and/or protein calorie malnutrition must discuss their diet with their physician and/or dietitian so that the cause of being underweight can be ascertained and treated. An impaired nutritional status is most commonly caused by:

◆ Active inflammatory disease

◆ Loss of appetite resulting from specific drug therapy

◆ Pain or depression

Weight loss and being underweight may contribute to the general feeling of malaise and fatigue characteristic of RA. Even though it uses up calories, exercise stimulates appetite and is an important component of therapy. Nutritional supplementation may be indicated.

Being overweight increases the stress on joints and therefore increases pain. In general, being overweight is caused by:

◆ Decreased physical activity

◆ Corticosteroid-induced hunger and altered metabolism

◆ Depression-induced overeating

Since being overweight is a national problem, you will be familiar with many commonly used strategies. Diets of the month published in popular magazines are usually a poor choice, because they tend to neglect your specific nutritional needs. It is important that you develop a sound eating plan and follow it to the best of your ability. Tips on how to maintain an adequate diet are discussed in this chapter.

DIETARY SUPPLEMENTS

Often, for a variety of reasons, you may be advised to supplement your regular diet with vitamins or minerals. Like foods and over-the-counter (OTC) medications, vitamin/mineral supplements have meaningful labels. Note that a typical multivitamin preparation supplies in excess of 100 percent of 17 micronutrients, the only exception being calcium, which is required in large amounts. Calcium is most easily available in dairy foods. Antacids also contain large amounts of calcium. You may supplement your dietary calcium intake with a suitable calcium supplement.

Many food supplements have been recommended for the treatment of RA. As you know, RA is a very changeable disease, and it is often difficult to know whether you feel better because of a dietary supplement or because of the cyclical nature the disease. Here is a survey of common, currently popular dietary supplements whose use may have some rational basis.

In 1999, Marcy O'Koon, the editor of *Arthritis Today,* the consumer magazine published by the Arthritis Foundation, visited a trade expo for dietary supplements at which more than 1,600 exhibitors plied their wares. (For details, see *Arthritis Today,* March–April 1999.) Best-sellers included herbs (garlic, ginseng, St. John's wort), minerals (from calcium to zinc), vitamins, and specialty supplements (glucosamine, melatonin, fish oils/cartilage, DHEA). Most of what was offered will end up at your local health food store. O'Koon advises her readers to be cautious shoppers. Her special recommendations include evaluating the knowledge of sales clerks (Do they believe all forms of arthritis are the same?), researching the product (books, Internet—you can reach the FDA at vm.cfsan. fda.gov), reading labels, trying only one preparation at a time, and, above all, informing your doctor. Report any adverse reactions promptly to your health care advisors.

The following nutritional supplements have been around for a number of years. Isabelle Dube, RD, CDN, Department of Food and Nutrition, HSS, writes in *Health Connection* (volume 9, number 1, Summer 2000): "These supplements are currently being studied and still lack clinical evidence to be prescribed for general use. Much is still unknown about possible drug interactions and side effects of nutritional supplements." Dube advises her readers to discuss the use of these supplements with their physician and points out that the FDA does not regulate these preparations. Like other authorities, Dube stresses that the listing of these supplements is not an endorsement or recommendation, and indeed some of these preparations may be harmful or interfere with the medications you are taking.

Chondroitin Sulfate

Often used in combination with glucosamine, chondroitin sulfate is supposed to reduce pain and stiffness. In the test tube it inhibits the breakdown of cartilage. The supplement has blood-thinning effects and may augment the blood-thinning action of drugs.

Fish Oils

Fish oils contain a high concentration of highly polyunsaturated fatty acids (PUFAs). In the body, these give rise to some of the prostaglandins, which are the precursors of the major immunomodulators that play a crucial role in generating/suppressing the inflammation characteristic of RA. Several studies suggest that fish oil supplementation decreases fatigue, joint tenderness, and morning stiffness. The use of fish oil capsules seems safe, but longer toxicity studies are required. A fishy smell and taste may accompany consumption of fish oils. These supplements may interact with other blood-thinning herbs or drugs. They also contain large amounts of vitamins A and D, which are stored in the body and are harmful when consumed in excess.

GLA Oils (Evening Primrose Oil, Borage Oils, Others)

These preparations provide highly unsaturated essential fatty acids that promote the release of anti-inflammatory precursors of "good" prostaglandins. Results so far are promising but require confirmation and long-term toxicity studies. These supplements may interact with other blood-thinning herbs or drugs.

Glucosamine

Most RA patients are aware of the excitement that surrounded the use of glucosamine with or without chondroitin sulfate. Both substances are building blocks of articular cartilage. Unfortunately, it is nearly impossible to "convince" an adult body to utilize externally supplied building blocks, and glucosamine is no exception. The drug(s), however, may decrease pain. Psychological factors may again play a role. Doyt Conn, M.D., the previous medical director of the Arthritis Foundation, believes that it is unlikely that these substances result in permanent improvement. Currently, the Arthritis Foundation cannot advise people to take these preparations. New research, however, will answer the question.

MEDICATIONS AND FOOD INTAKE FOR PATIENTS WITH RA

Medications—whether taken for RA or for other reasons—can affect nutrient absorption in several ways:

- By binding to specific nutrients in food, thereby preventing the body from utilizing it.
- By promoting blood loss from the gastrointestinal tract, thereby increasing the requirement for iron and folic acid.
- By interfering with the absorption (vitamin B_{12}) or the excretion of specific vitamins, thereby promoting specific vitamin deficiencies.
- By interfering with electrolyte balance (sodium and potassium concentration in body fluids), thereby promoting dehydration or fluid retention. This may necessitate the manipulation of electrolyte intake.
- By destroying the intestinal flora that produces vitamin K that is essential for blood coagulation.
- By affecting taste and appetite, which may affect proper food intake.

Table 11–5 lists the nutritional impact of some relevant medications. The problems, however, should be discussed with your physician, pharmacist, and/or dietitian.

TABLE 11-5. Possible Nutritional Effects of Some Drugs
Used for the Treatment of RA

Nonsteroidal Anti-Inflammatory Drugs		
Medication	**Possible Effect**	**Remedy**
NSAIDs such as aspirin, ibuprofen, others	Stomach irritation, ulcers, iron and folate deficiency	Always take with food and never on an empty stomach.

DMARDs, Cytotoxic Agents

Since cytotoxic agents destroy the fast-growing cells that form the mucous membranes of the intestine, these drugs often irritate the mouth, stomach, and gut, causing sores, cracks, and fissures. They may interfere with food intake. Cytotoxic agents may also cause nausea and/or vomiting. All cytotoxic agents are immunosuppressive and promote bacterial overgrowth of the mouth and GI tract (candida, others). Scrupulous mouth care including topical or systemic antimicrobial agents may be prescribed.

Medication	**Possible Effect**	**Remedy**
Azathioprine	Nausea, vomiting, diarrhea, mouth sores	Take medication with meals or in divided dosage. If necessary, discuss dosage reduction with your physician.
Cyclophosphamide	Nausea, vomiting, decreased appetite	Drink large amounts of fluid.
Cyclosporine	Nausea, vomiting, diarrhea, constipation, loss of appetite, cramps, overgrown gums, irritated stomach, ulcers	Divide dose to lessen side effects. Avoid grapefruit juice.
Leflunomide	Diarrhea, metallic taste	Divide dose to lessen side effects.
Methotrexate	Anorexia and nausea, especially during the 24 hours after dosing	Side effects may decrease with administration of folic acid.

Miscellaneous Agents		
Medication	**Possible Effect**	**Remedy**
Gold	Metallic taste, GI upset, nausea, vomiting, diarrhea, cramps	Maintain adequate food intake. Side effects decrease with usage.

TABLE II-5. *(continued)*

Medication	Possible Effect	Remedy
Hydroxychloroquine	Cramps, GI upset, nausea, vomiting	A temporary reduction in dosage may help if symptoms are excessive.
Penicillamine	Altered taste, nausea, vomiting, loss of appetite, reactivation of ulcers, mouth ulcers	Take drug on empty stomach 1 hour before or 2 hours after meals. Maintain adequate food intake. Supplement vitamin B_6.
Sulfasalazine	Loss of appetite, vomiting, nausea; impairs absorption of folic acid and may complex with iron	Take with food to reduce GI upset. Supplement folic acid and vitamin B_6. Avoid iron supplementation.

Drugs used to treat other medical conditions (hypertension, diabetes, infections), as well as sleeping pills, cathartic medications, antacids, and alcohol, may also affect nutrient utilization. Some of these effects are listed below:

Medication	Possible Effect
Alcohol	Malabsorption of folic acid and vitamin B_{12}
Antacids	Phosphate depletion, muscle weakness, vitamin D deficiency
Antidiabetics (oral)	Impair absorption of vitamin B_{12}
Anti-infective	Wipe out intestinal flora and decrease synthesis of vitamin K
Cathartics	Decrease nutrient absorption
Contraceptives (oral)	Deplete folic acid and vitamin B_6
Diuretics	Potassium depletion
Mineral oil	Interferes with the absorption of fat-soluble vitamins D, E, K, and carotene
Neomycin	Impairs absorption of vitamin B_{12}
Phenobarbital	Folate deficiency
Phenothiazine, tricyclic antidepressants	Stimulate appetite, increase food intake, cause weight gain

EATING HEALTHILY
DURING CORTICOSTEROID THERAPY

"I want to rip into a side of beef, devour an entire cheesecake, down a quart of Ben and Jerry's, crunch a bag of Doritos," says Eugenia Zuckerman, the flutist who we met in Chapter 9. "I always walk around half starved," says Samantha F., who we met in Chapter 1. "I am accustomed to controlling my food intake," says Ursula B., a longstanding diabetic. "Still, it was extremely difficult to cope with the ravenous hunger caused by the steroids."

As anyone who has experienced corticosteroid therapy knows, these hormones increase the body's craving for food, sometimes grossly altering a person's looks. In a way, this is not surprising. The glucocorticosteroid hormones, of which prednisone is a synthetic variety, play a major role in the manner in which the body transforms food into energy. The corticosteroids seem to switch the body into a more economical way of storing nutrients. Like animals during hibernation, corticosteroids slow the metabolism and promote fat storage. The drugs also increase blood glucose and affect salt metabolism. The latter, in turn, promotes fluid retention.

Curtailing food intake while on corticosteroid therapy is tremendously difficult. In addition to stimulating appetite, these drugs increase a person's emotional fragility, and eating is a common way of relieving tension.

The effort is nevertheless worthwhile. The ways of eating healthily while on corticosteroids do not differ markedly from any other weight-control plan, except that you should pay close attention to the altered physiological effects of these drugs. Here are a few suggestions.

What Not to Eat

Limit salt intake. Salt promotes fluid retention. It is important to avoid salting food during cooking or at the table. At first, such a bland diet may be unpleasant, but within a number of months your taste buds will be used to it. Remember the following tips:

◆ Do not salt food when cooking at home.

◆ Today many restaurants cater to clients with special dietary requirements. Make sure you specify "no salt."

- Read food labels to ensure that cans and other packaged foods are salt-free.

- Buy no-salt-added dairy products.

- Avoid buying prepared meats, herring, pickles, olives, and pretzels.

Limit the intake of concentrated carbohydrates (simple sugars) because elevated blood glucose levels can be one of the side effects of corticosteroid therapy. Avoid desserts and sweets.

Limit the consumption of fats. Like sweets, many fatty foods simply supply calories and contribute few useful nutrients such as protein, minerals, and vitamins to your diet.

What to Eat

If you are always hungry, it is especially important to plan what you are actually going to eat. Food should be pleasing; otherwise, the resolve to limit calories will vanish.

Preparing tasty low-calorie food is time-consuming. When your RA is active, you may not have the energy to fuss in the kitchen. Rely on prepared items such as frozen food (vegetables), no-salt soups, and canned tuna fish in water.

Modern kitchen appliances will enable you to prepare tasty, low-calorie foods without much effort or cleanup. A microwave bakes a potato in 8 minutes and steams fish in 3. A blender makes a "smoothie" in 2 minutes.

Three meals a day are good, though some people are less hungry when they have more frequent, smaller meals.

Your meals should be rich in nutrients. Select dairy foods for calcium, fruits and vegetables for vitamins and minerals, and high-quality protein foods. Good food choices include grilled meats and fish, legumes, tofu, and cottage cheese.

Snacking is an important aspect of being able to stay on a diet when hungry. When developing your meal plan, allow for healthy snacks. Table 11–6 presents some suggestions.

TABLE 11-6. Healthy Snacks

Buttermilk/skim milk smoothie: Blend 8 ounces of milk, one banana, ice, and perhaps an artificial sweetener.

Rice crackers

Fresh fruit

Frozen banana

Celery sticks, carrots, radishes, scallions

Nonfat yogurt with aspartame and mashed-up fruit

Hard-boiled egg

12

Exercise, Physical Therapy, and RA

Appropriate exercise is one of the most important aspects of therapy. This chapter provides an in-depth overview of therapeutic and recreational exercises, as well as tips on how to develop, maintain, and enjoy these activities.

"You are incredible," Todd Cronin, a physical therapist (PT) on the staff of the Hospital for Special Surgery (HSS), told his audience. "Some of you have been operated on twenty different times," Cronin continued, "and yet, when you come for a session of physical therapy, you smile, do whatever is necessary to stay functional, and never complain."

Mr. Cronin was addressing 20 or so men and women who belonged to the HSS support group, Living with RA, led by Adina Batterman. (We'll meet the group more extensively in Chapter 13.) The topic of the day was "The Benefits of Physical Therapy and Exercise."

The majority of the attendees were veteran RA sufferers. Some have had the disease since childhood; for others, the onset was more recent. Most had come to the meeting unaided, some used canes, and one woman arrived in a wheelchair pushed by an attendant. Most patients were middle-aged. Even though many had longstanding RA, they had come because they wanted to learn more about how to live well by controlling their disease.

How Exercise Can Benefit Patients with RA

The use of exercise to treat people suffering from RA is rather new. Years ago, rheumatologists ordered strict bed rest for RA sufferers, which often resulted in pretzel-like deformations and thin bones. Today, everybody realizes that the optimal balance of both rest and exercise plays a major role in RA treatment. Specifically, the function of exercise is to:

◆ Improve joint function by maintaining, improving, and/or increasing range of motion, overall flexibility, joint mechanics, muscular support of joints, strength, and stability

◆ Decrease pain, fatigue, and morning stiffness

◆ Decrease depression

◆ Maintain joint protection

◆ Improve overall physical status and conditioning

◆ Play an active role in disease control and avoidance of deformity

Using Your Joints

A healthy joint is totally dependent on its muscle tissue. Muscle tone, in turn, is a function of use. The muscles of a limb encased in a cast atrophy rapidly. For those without joint impairment, a normal lifestyle provides enough exercise to keep muscles in reasonable shape.

Not using a joint enough, however, is a major problem for those with RA. Pain and the associated avoidance of using the painful joint has a cascade effect. Disuse leads to the loss of muscle tissue, and ultimately increased joint deterioration. One of the goals of physical therapy is to prevent this loss and to ensure that muscles remain mobile, strong, stretched, functional, and properly aligned.

Exercise also relieves pain. We automatically wiggle a foot that has fallen asleep. Cats and dogs stretch after their naps, and we, too, feel good stretching in bed before getting up.

Exercise for RA is much more formal than stretching in bed. Today, exercise should be a regular component of your treatment plan. No rheumatologist or orthopedic surgeon will ever let you forget it. People who have undergone total joint replacement will attest to the fact that long before they recovered from the traumatic effects of the surgery they were made to walk, flex their shoulders, or stand to test their new knees. The health professional in charge of these exercises is the physical therapist.

As the healing professions go, physical therapy is relatively young. Its professional beginnings date from the 1950s when polio was at its height and health professionals tried to rehabilitate the paralyzed. Like Todd Cronin, most physical therapists are upbeat, cheerful, trim, and truly devoted to the well-being of their patients. "We get to know our patients better than the doctor does," Cronin told his audience at HSS. Indeed, many patients love their physical therapists because of their "can-do" attitude.

In addition to exercises, physical therapists provide canes and other assistive devices, administer heat treatments and transcutaneous nerve stimulation (TENS), and, if you are lucky, give you a massage (see Chapter 14).

The activities of the physical therapist may overlap with those of the occupational therapist (see Chapter 13).

ASSESSMENT

Exercise must be carefully prescribed. Like medications, too much, too little, too soon, or the wrong kind may do more harm than good. The physician writes the initial exercise prescription. The exact terms of the prescription, however, are usually vague and may read something like: gluteal and quad (quadriceps) strengthening, or increase ROM of shoulder. The physical therapist will fill in the all-important functional details.

To begin with, the physical therapist will make his or her own assessment. During the initial session, the PT will evaluate your health by carefully reviewing your medical history and evaluating your physical status. You will be asked to bend your joints (called *active range of motion*) and then the therapist will bend them (called *passive range of motion*).

Ambulatory patients will be directed to walk, stand, sit, and get up from a chair. You will be asked to bend, lift your arms above your head, touch your buttocks with your heel, and lock your elbows.

Your overall health, including cardiovascular fitness, will be evaluated. The activity of the disease will be carefully assessed. Since inflamed joints should not be exercised, there often is a thin line between too much exercise and too little.

The physical therapist will pay careful attention to what you can or cannot do. This is a functional assessment. Typical questions are: Can you dress yourself? How far can you walk? Can you reach up and get stuff from the top shelf of the closet? Can you pick things up from the floor? Can you hook your bra? Can you take care of your personal needs?

Thereafter, treatment goals will be established. After surgery, or after a severe flare, these goals may be as seemingly small as getting out of bed or negotiating a flight of stairs; sometime, however, the goals are as major as walking half a mile.

Physical therapists will help and encourage you to achieve and exceed these goals. A good physical therapist will provide you with real-istic expectations. Do not hope to run a marathon when RA is attacking your hips and knees. "Your joints will have good days and bad days," Todd Cronin cautions his audience at HSS. "On good days, do a little more; on bad days, do fewer repetitions."

As with all the other aspects of care, you, the patient, will ultimately be responsible for doing the exercises on your own that are prescribed by your physical therapist. You will be given clear, simple instructions, but might still be confused. "We try to follow the KISS principle," Todd Cronin joked. When asked what he meant, Cronin explained that KISS stands for "Keep It Simple, Stupid." You can always ask for a refresher course.

TYPES OF EXERCISES USED FOR RA

Exercises are subdivided into range of motion (ROM) and stretching exercises, which maintain joint flexibility, and strengthening exercises, which maintain and augment muscle tone. Recreational exercises, which improve overall health and fitness, are also crucial for people suffering from RA.

The goal of range of motion exercises is to maintain and/or restore the maximum movement in a particular joint. To this end, the joint is moved (rotated, bent) in all directions as far as it will comfortably go.

The range of motion exercises are further subdivided into passive ROM exercises during which the therapist rotates or flexes your joint as far as it will go and active ROM exercises during which the joint is moved with some assistance supplied either by the therapist (active assisted) or yourself (active). Stretching is similar to ROM exercises except that the joint is stretched a bit beyond its comfortable range. Range of motion and stretching exercises should make you feel good and relieve pain and stiffness. As a rule, patients are instructed to do their ROM exercises once or twice daily and repeat each exercise 5 to 10 times.

Strengthening exercises will strengthen the muscles surrounding the joint, thereby improving joint movement, alignment, and function, as well as decreasing fatigue and pain. Two types of strengthening exercises are used for people with RA: isometric exercises and isotonic exercises.

During isometric (static) exercises, the muscles surrounding the joint are tightened without moving the joint. One example is tightening your buttocks while sitting on a chair. These exercises are particularly useful for painful joints.

During isotonic (dynamic) exercises, muscles are moved and tightened against resistance such as a light weight or your own body. Initially, isometric exercises should be done under the supervision of a therapist. Examples are extending your leg while sitting and opening your arms while stretching a rubber exercise band.

Figure 12–1 illustrates commonly used ROM and strengthening exercises. Your therapist may provide you with a different set of exercises.

The Exercise Prescription and Performance

Exercise prescriptions for people suffering from RA are highly individualized and depend both on the activity of the disease and the joints affected. The prescription specifies both the type of exercise to do and the number of times it should be done (repetitions).

Initially, your physical therapist will watch you perform the exercises; then you will be on your own. It is highly desirable that every so often the therapist recheck your performance. Given the restrictions imposed by managed care plans, this is not always feasible. A phone call or a fax, however, may be sufficient in some situations.

Develop a routine for doing your exercises. Schedule them as faithfully as you do your meals. Select a specific place and time for doing them. You may wish to do them with music, while watching a favorite television program, or with an exercise tape. Exercise for 20 to 30 minutes at a time if this is possible.

Exercise when you hurt least. If necessary, exercise when the effect of your medications is at its maximum.

Remember that "cold" muscles won't stretch. It may help you to precede your exercises with a hot shower or bath. You can also relax tight muscles with a warm, moist towel.

Start your exercise sessions by stretching every part of your body and then warm up with ROM exercises. Terminate by "cooling down."

FIGURE 12-1. Sample ROM and Stretch Exercises. *Exercises 12-1a–r from the* Manual of Rheumatology and Outpatient Orthopedic Disorders, *3rd ed. by Stephen Paget, Paul Pellici, and John F. Beary III. Lippincott, Williams & Wilkins. The exercises were designed by Sandy B. Ganz and Louis Harris.*

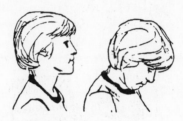

12-1-a. Neck flexion. Sitting or standing with your back straight, bend your head forward and tuck your chin in toward your chest.

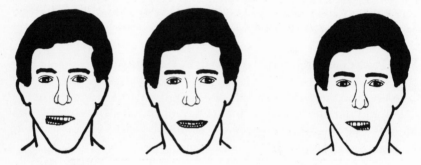

12-1-b. Lateral jaw excursion. Smile so that your bottom and top teeth are touching. Move your mouth from right to left.

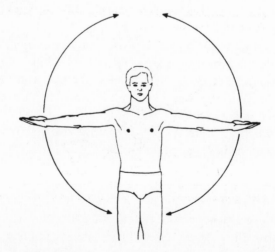

12-1-c. Arm rotation. Stand with your arms extended at your side, palms facing front. Rotate your arms forward in a circle. Reverse arms.

FIGURE 12-1. *(continued)*

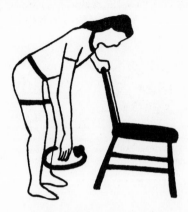

12-1-d. Pendulum exercises. Stand holding onto a sturdy chair with your uninvolved arm. Bend forward at the waist and bend your knees to help protect your back. Let the arm hang limp. Keep the shoulder relaxed and use body motion to swing your arm in a circle.

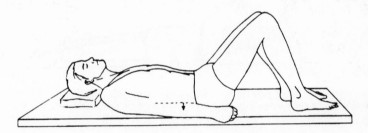

12-1-e. Back. Lying on your back with knees bent, press the small of your back into the bed or floor. Tighten your abdominal and buttock muscles.

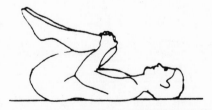

12-1-f. Knees to chest. Lying on your back, slowly bring both knees up to your chest.

FIGURE 12-1. *(continued)*

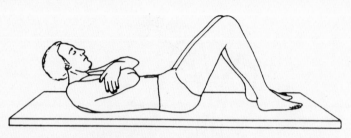

12-1-g. Partial sit-ups. Lie on your back with your knees bent and arms crossed. With your chin tucked, slowly lift your head and shoulders toward your knees.

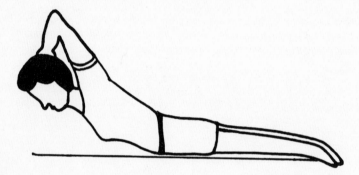

12-1-h. Lift—prone. Lie on your stomach with a pillow under your abdomen. Place your hands behind your head. Raise your head and chest.

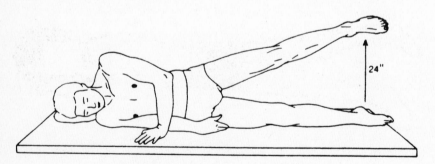

12-1-i. Leg lifts. Lie on your side. Use your lower leg to keep your balance. Keep your top leg straight. Raise it to the ceiling in line with your body. Lower it slowly.

FIGURE 12-1. *(continued)*

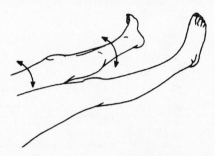

12-1-j. Hip, external rotation. Lie on your back with your legs straight. Roll your leg outward.

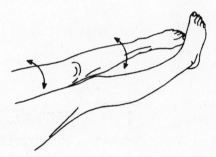

12-1-k. Hip, internal rotation. Lie on your back with your legs straight. Roll your leg inward.

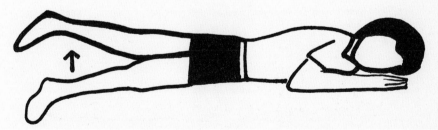

12-1-l. Prone hip extension. Lie on your stomach with both legs straight. Lift your legs, one at a time, toward the ceiling, keeping your knees straight. Slowly lower your leg.

FIGURE 12-1. *(continued)*

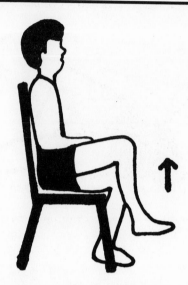

12-1-m. Hip flexion. Sit on a chair with both feet flat on the floor. Raise one knee toward your chest as high as possible.

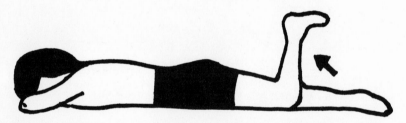

12-1-n. Knee flexion—prone. Lie on your stomach with both legs straight. Bend your knees one at a time as far as possible.

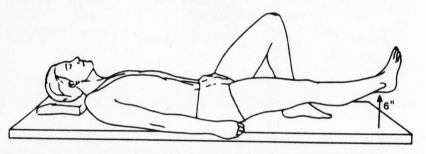

12-1-o. Knee strengthening. Lie on your back with one leg bent, the other straight. Tighten the thigh muscles of the straight leg, slowly lift, and lower. Change.

FIGURE 12-1. (continued)

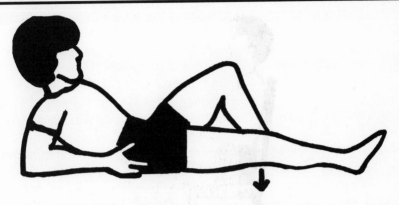

12-1-p. Quad set. Half-sit with one leg straight, one bent. Tighten the muscles on top of the thigh.

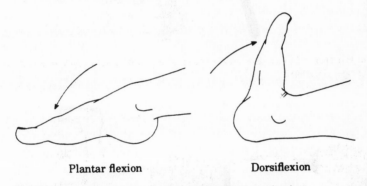

Plantar flexion   Dorsiflexion

12-1-q. Ankle flexion. Point toes down, then bring them toward your head.

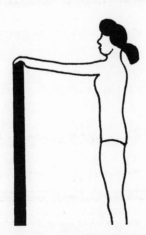

12-1-r. Heel cord stretch. Stand with the ball of the foot on a book. Hold onto a counter or firm surface. Try to place your heels on the floor. Gently lean forward, keeping your knees straight. Hold, then stand on toes. Return to starting position. Do both feet together or alternate.

Exercise and Disease Activity

RA presents you with a dilemma. Everyone on your health care team stresses that you must exercise. Yet, they will also caution you not to exercise an actively inflamed joint. As with other aspects of your treatment, you will have to decide when and how much to exercise.

During acute disease and flares: Use pain as your guide. Try to maintain the range of motion of the affected joints. Gently perform ROM and isometric (tightening) exercises. Do only a few repetitions. Increase rest periods.

During moderately active disease: Increase ROM and strengthening exercises slowly. As always, use pain as your guide and cut back if you notice that your joints get worse (more pain, swelling, or increased warmth). Be aware that you may feel better one day and worse the next, or that even the same joint on the other side may behave differently. Try returning to fitness activity (swimming, aquatic exercises).

During chronic, nonactive RA: Return to your usual exercise regimen.

THE SURGEON GENERAL'S RECOMMENDATIONS

Exercise, as we understand it today, is a new phenomenon. Past generations worked on the farm. Children walked or biked to school, women scrubbed the floors, and men chopped wood. With the development of technology, by the 1950s it became evident that as a nation we were physically unfit and increasingly obese. The Surgeon General, other government agencies, health columnists, and physicians have become adamant about exercise. They have been somewhat successful. Our parks are full of runners and bikers, health clubs are a growth industry, and wearing the latest sneakers is a status symbol. The results have been positive. Life expectancy has lengthened, though it is hard to know whether the improvement is due to diet, better drugs, surgery, and/or exercise.

As you well know, physical activity is both crucial and difficult for people suffering from RA. However, since it is such an important component of care for patients, it was the subject of a daylong meeting organized by the Association of Rheumatology Health Professionals (ARHP) in 1997.

To begin, Marion A. Minor, PT, Ph.D., reviewed the overall findings and recommendations of the Surgeon General's report on "Physical Activity and Health" (see Table 12–1). This summary highlights the aspects of greatest significance for people suffering from musculoskeletal diseases.

TABLE 12-1. Highlights from "Physical Activity and Health: Report of the Surgeon General"

1. For better health, physical activity should be performed regularly and include a minimum of moderate-intensity activity on most days of the week.

2. Cardiovascular fitness* should be supplemented with strengthening exercises at least twice a week to improve musculoskeletal health, maintain independence, and reduce risk of falls.

3. Physical activity has beneficial effects for all ages on cardiovascular, musculoskeletal, metabolic, endocrine, and immune system function. Benefits disappear within 2 to 8 months of insufficient physical therapy.

4. Moderate levels of physical activity (compared to sedentary habits) are associated with lower mortality rates in both younger and older adults.

5. Regular physical activity decreases cardiovascular disease, prevents/reduces hypertension, and is associated with a decreased risk of colon cancer, adult-onset diabetes, and obesity.

6. Regular moderately intense physical activity is necessary to maintain muscle strength, joint structure, and function. Such exercise may be beneficial to people suffering from arthritis. It is unclear whether exercise can reduce the accelerated bone loss in postmenopausal women in the absence of estrogen replacement therapy.

7. Physical activity relieves symptoms of depression and anxiety, and improves mood and health-related quality of life, particularly in those compromised by poor health.

8. Only about 22 percent of adults in the United States engage in regular sustained physical activity of any intensity. Most popular adult physical activities are walking and gardening/yard work.

9. Consistent influences on physical activity patterns include self-efficacy, enjoyment, social support, belief in benefits of exercise, and lack of perceived barriers.

*In this context, *cardiovascular* and *cardiorespiratory* refer to activities that use the large muscles of the body that control the function of the heart and lungs, respectively.

Source: Adapted from Marion A. Minor, PT, Ph.D. From *New Approaches to Physical Activities for People with Rheumatic Diseases*. Presented at Physical Activity as a Lifestyle, Not Just Therapy, ARHP Clinical Focus Course, Washington, DC, 1997.

We have already reviewed the therapeutic exercises used to maintain joint function and overall muscle tone. These activities, however, are not sufficient to maintain overall fitness. To fulfill the Surgeon General's recommendations, people with RA must also do aerobic exercises. These exercises strengthen the large muscles of the body that work the heart and lungs. Typical aerobic activities include walking, swimming, golf, and bicycling, as well as daily activities such as mopping the floor, gardening, and raking leaves.

Previously, it had been assumed that such aerobic conditioning required 20 minutes of sustained exercise performed three times per week. This prolonged effort might exceed the capabilities of people suffering from RA. Fortunately, however, exercise physiologists discovered that the 20-minute session can be broken up into smaller segments such as two 10-minute sessions or even four 5-minute ones. This finding is good news for people with limited capabilities.

Many of these activities present a challenge for people suffering from RA. As usual, you must make an extra effort to find an aerobic activity that you like and can do. As always, whether you can participate in a particular sport depends on the extent of your arthritis and on which part of your body is affected. Table 12–2 lists overall information on what exercises might be suitable.

RECREATIONAL ACTIVITY FOR PEOPLE SUFFERING FROM RA

Many common recreational activities can be adapted to people suffering from RA. As always, you must use pain as your guide and distinguish between being simply tired from your exercises and from joint overuse.

A few pertinent facts about sports and recreational activities are explained in this chapter. The Arthritis Foundation provides booklets on

TABLE 12-2. Activities Suitable for People Suffering from RA

If the Rheumatoid Arthritis Affects	You Can
Upper extremities (shoulders, elbows, hands)	Swim, do aquatic exercises, walk, cross-country ski
Back, spine	Swim, do aquatic exercises
Lower extremities (hips, knees, ankles, feet)	Swim, do aquatic exercises, row, golf, use a stationary bicycle, canoe, water running.

Source: From *The Columbia-Presbyterian Osteoarthritis Handbook*, Ronald P. Grelsemar and Suzanne Loebl, eds. Macmillan, 1996, 1997.

some specific activities (golf, gardening, aquatics). Relevant articles are regularly published in *Arthritis Today*. *The Sports Injury Handbook* by Allan M. Levy and Mark L. Fuerst (John Wiley) is also useful. *The Guide for Independent Living* is full of useful gadgets that can help you in your chosen activity. As always, discuss your planned activity with your physician or physical therapist.

Participating in recreational exercise or sports is an excellent way of improving physical fitness and mental attitude. Such activities, however, must be pleasurable. Don't invest in expensive golf equipment if you can't hit a ball or join a health club if you hate exercising indoors surrounded by others. All physical activity must be preceded by a warm-up session—a set of stretching exercises will do—and conclude with a cooldown session—again, stretching will do.

One more tip: Take pain-relieving medication before exercising.

Water Exercises

For patients suffering from arthritis, water is a blessing. Sore muscles are buoyed and soothed by water. Stiff limbs relax and can be moved, tender joints feel normal, and the joy of movement returns.

Aquatics are extremely beneficial. There are many different ways of enjoying water. You may swim, walk in the water, or do your own aquatics.

Many people love the aquatic classes organized by the Arthritis Foundation. In addition to exercise, these classes offer companionship. Call your local chapter of the Arthritis Foundation for information. Most often, these classes are taught at the local Y.

In addition, or instead, you may prefer exercising on your own. The "Water Exercise, Pools, Spas and Arthritis" booklet (free from the Arthritis Foundation) illustrates exercises to do in the water, including leg swings (hip flexion), knee lifts, calf stretches, side bends, hand and finger exercises, and much more.

You may prefer swimming, which stretches and strengthens muscles and provides overall conditioning. You may have to modify your strokes. If your neck hurts when you turn it to breathe out during the crawl, lift it. If that is too much motion, swim with a mask and a snorkel. If your knees mind the frog kick, do the butterfly kick. Persevere—it is worth it.

Even though it may seem easy, exercising in water appropriately strengthens muscles and increases range of motion. Start every exercise session with a few minutes of warm-ups and conclude with a cool-down.

Spas and Hot Tubs

If you swim at a health club, you may have access to a hot tub or sauna. Most patients feel better after a session of warm, moist heat—so good in fact that those who can afford it may purchase a whirlpool for home use.

Exercise Tapes

Many people love exercising while listening to or viewing an exercise tape. A few of the recommended tapes are listed in Table 12-3, but availability changes. As always, use pain as your guide when using these tapes.[1]

Walking

Walking may be the best overall exercise for people suffering from RA. According to Marion A. Minor and Victoria Gall, physical therapists and exercise specialists, "Walking can help condition heart and lungs, strengthen bones and muscles, relieve tension, control weight, and improve energy and mood. Walking is easy, inexpensive, safe, and accessible. You can walk by yourself or with company, and you can take your exercise with you wherever you go." The experts present some suggestions on how to walk in spite of arthritis in Table 12-4.

Tennis

People with severe RA will shudder at the thought of hopping around a tennis court. Those with mild disease may be able to continue cautiously, especially if they switch to doubles. Ping-Pong may also be an alternative.

Health Clubs

You may benefit from joining a health club, whose fee is often covered, at least partially, by your health insurance. First of all, your health club provides companionship. Its staff usually includes physical trainers who instruct you on how to use exercise machines. Be sure to inform them

---

[1] These tapes were suggested by K. F. Haralson and Michele Boutaugh at the ARHP Clinical Focus Course: Physical Activity as a Lifestyle, Not Just Therapy, Washington, DC, 1997.

TABLE 12-3. Exercise Tapes for People with Arthritis

1. *People with Arthritis Can Exercise (PACE), Level 1 and Level 2:* PACE Level 1 helps people with arthritis to keep moving and stay active. Includes gentle stretching, strengthening, and fitness exercises. PACE Level 2 has a longer endurance-building segment. Order by phone 1-800-207-8633 or by mail from Arthritis Foundation Fulfillment Center, P.O. Box 6996, Alpharetta, GA 30009–6996.

2. *Pathways to Better Living with Arthritis and Related Conditions:* Includes stretches, strengthening exercises, aerobics, as well as breathing and relaxation techniques. Also available in Spanish. Same ordering information as for number 1. Also, 800-366-6038, or www.mobilitylt.com.

3. *Pathways Exercise Video for People with Limited Mobility:* Same ordering information as for number 2.

4. *Arthritis Foundation Pool Exercise Programs:* Same ordering information as for number 1.

5. *Good Moves for Every Body* and *Good Moves 2:* Tapes are designed for people with arthritis and/or those not familiar with exercise. *Good Moves 1* is a three-part program of warm-up exercises for flexibility, low-impact aerobics, aerobic dance, and five 4-minute routines. *Good Moves 2* is a low-intensity exercise program containing two 20-minute sessions. Order from Arthritis Center Exercise Video, MA427, Health Service Center, University of Missouri, Columbia, MO 65211.

6. *ROM Dance Videotapes (3):* Each *ROM Dance* videotape includes step-by-step instructions for range-of-motion exercises to be done to music and the reading of light verse. The videos also include a guided relaxation session. The three available versions are: *The ROM Dance in Sunlight, The ROM Dance in Moonlight,* and *The ROM Dance: Seated Version.* Order from 1-800-488-4940 or ROM Dance, P.O. Box 3332, Madison, WI 53704.

of your physical limitations. If there is a question about your intended activities, ask your physician or physical therapist. Finally, most health clubs organize exercise classes. You may not be able to take aerobics classes, but there are many classes that may be perfectly suitable for you (yoga, stretch classes, stay-fit for seniors), especially when you modify the activities to suit your needs.

Exercise Machines

Because exercise machines can be adapted to people suffering from chronic disease, their use is highly recommended. Exercise machines can be used in the gym or purchased for home use.

TABLE 12-4. Walking for People Suffering from Arthritis

Is walking for you? Determine whether you can walk for 10 minutes without increasing your pain or discomfort. If you can, proceed.

Choose your ground. Walk on flat, level surfaces. Hills, uneven ground, soft earth, sand, or gravel are hard work. Use fitness trails, shopping malls, school tracks, and streets with sidewalks.

Wear supportive shoes in good repair. Athletic and walking shoes have better shock absorption and support than leather-soled shoes. Insoles and heel cups of shock-absorbing material can be used for comfort.

Begin and end with a stroll. Stroll for 3 to 5 minutes to prepare your muscles for a brisker walk, and finish up with the same slow stroll.

Set your own pace. It takes practice to find a walking speed that is good for you. Start slowly and increase your pace to slightly above your normal walking speed. Can you sing out loud or talk without getting out of breath? Choose a pace that you think you could maintain for 15 minutes. Remember that walking faster puts more stress on your knees. Use a cane to decrease stress on your weight-bearing joints if necessary.

Arms and legs together. The conditioning effect of walking also depends on the length of your stride and the swing of your arms. Increasing either of these will increase the effectiveness of the workout.

Time and distance: How much to do? It is often more enjoyable and satisfying to walk for a certain period of time rather than for a specific distance. Most often, you can complete a time goal even when you need to walk more slowly or combine periods of brisk walking with slow ones and resting. Initially keep your walking time to 10 or 20 minutes, and gradually increase it to 30.

Source: Adapted from Minor and Gall presentation at Physical Activity as a Lifestyle, Not Just Therapy, ARHP Clinical Focus Course, Washington, DC, 1997.

The stationary bicycle is the most widely used exercise machine. Be sure to choose a model in which the tension can be adjusted. The machine is ideal for those suffering from RA of the upper extremities. Those with hip and knee involvement should use caution.

When mastered, skiing machines provide weight-bearing, rhythmic motion of the legs and arms, thereby providing excellent aerobic conditioning. Because your feet stay put, the impact on the weight-bearing joints is much less that that associated with treadmills.

Rowing machines, which are non-weight-bearing, provide excellent overall conditioning. Rowing entails bending of the hips and knees, which may be contraindicated for people suffering from RA of the weight-bearing joints.

Since the walking speed of treadmills can be adjusted, this weight-bearing exercise machine is suitable for many people suffering from RA.

Exercise with weight-lifting machines is designed to strengthen individual groups of muscles. In general, they must be used with great caution by people suffering from inflamed, impaired joints.

Exercises for Mind and Body

Physical activities that combine exercise with relaxation are very helpful for patients suffering from RA. It takes patience and determination to learn these techniques, and they are not everyone's cup of tea. The relaxation they induce is, however, quite extraordinary.

The best known of these techniques are yoga, the Alexander technique, and t'ai chi. It is usual to begin practicing these exercises in a group. Later, you can adapt them for use at home. You probably will have to adapt the exercises according to your particular impairment.

Yoga emphasizes stretching, deep breathing, and relaxation. The Alexander technique emphasizes posture and body alignment and enhances sensory awareness. T'ai chi, reputed to be 5,000 years old, originally was a form of martial art. Today, the slow, gentle movements are used to induce relaxation.

MAINTAINING YOUR EXERCISE PROGRAM

For most people, it is difficult to maintain an exercise program. Here are a few pointers:

- Keep an exercise diary.
- Choose a recreational activity you really like.
- Keep it simple. You will rarely exercise if it takes a long time to get to the gym or swimming pool.
- Exercise with friends.
- Exercise while you listen to a book on tape or watch TV.
- Vary your exercise routine
- Reward yourself when you have accomplished your exercise goals or done the best you could.

13

Occupational Therapy and RA of the Hands

———◆«◉»◆———

This chapter reviews ways of protecting joints from the destructive impact of RA. Special emphasis is placed on the small, vulnerable joints of the hands.

As Dr. Charles Christian, who for 25 years was physician-in-chief of the Hospital for Special Surgery, looked into the waiting room, he saw Mrs. Cooper (not her real name) knitting away at a furious rate. Dr. Christian was surprised. Mrs. Cooper suffered from longstanding RA and her hands were "a mess." Yet, like many other patients, she willed her distorted fingers to perform intricate tasks.

RA forces you to become a problem-solving expert. Auguste Renoir, the master Impressionist whose paintings are a celebration of life, suffered from severe RA during the last decades of his life. Most days, however, he asked a member of his household to strap a brush to his painful hand and went about producing his voluptuous images of women, flowers, and landscapes.

Even though patients are good at overcoming handicaps, they do even better when helped by an occupational therapist, the professional who specializes in teaching patients to manage difficult tasks and/or to do these tasks in a less harmful, more efficient, and convenient way.

There is overlap between occupational therapy and physical therapy. Traditionally, occupational therapists focus on restoring function of the small joints and on restoring function of the hands, while physical therapists are more concerned with larger joints.

ASSESSMENT

Evaluation always precedes treatment. However, instead of asking their clients what they cannot do, occupational therapists ask what they can do. When seeing an occupational therapist, be prepared to answer innumerable questions about *activities of daily living* (ADL). Here are some typical questions asked during a functional assessment:

Personal hygiene: Can you comb your hair? Can you turn the faucet, squeeze out toothpaste, brush your teeth, perform toileting, shave, cut your toenails, apply makeup? Can you open the vials and bottles your medicines come in?

Dressing: Can you dress and undress yourself? Can you put on socks, stockings, and pantyhose, pull up zippers, button buttons, put on an overcoat?

Cooking: Do you find it difficult to handle heavy objects such as pots and pans? Do you have trouble turning faucets, chopping and peeling vegetables, tearing open frozen food packages, opening cans, milk containers, and water bottles?

Eating: Can you cut your meat? Can you pick up a cup by its handle?

Housecleaning: Do you have trouble bending down? Can you handle a vacuum cleaner? Can you manage to turn the knobs on your washing machine?

Driving: Do you have trouble opening the car door or turning the ignition key?

Reading, writing, playing cards: Can you hold a pencil or pen? Can you turn the pages of a book? Can you handle playing cards?

In addition to a functional assessment, the occupational therapist will also evaluate pain, cosmetic appearance, the function and mechanics of joint actions, and anatomy. An in-depth evaluation requires specialized instruments including a goniometer (angle-measuring device), dynamometer, pinch gauge, ruler, sensory testing monofilaments, two-point discrimination compass, familiar objects to evaluate tactile (touch) identification, and cylinders of various sizes to measure the effectiveness of your grasp. Today, some institutions use the manual upper limb exerciser, which is discussed in this chapter.

ANATOMY OF THE HAND

"It is in the human hand," wrote the British anatomist Sir Charles Bell in 1833, "that we perceive the consummation of all; perfection, as an instrument. This superiority consists in its combination of strength, with variety, extent, and rapidity of motion . . . and the sensibility, which adapt it for holding, pulling, spinning, and constructing; with the hands the laborer supports a family, the parent loves and cares for a baby, the musician plays a sonata, the blind 'read,' and the deaf 'talk.' "

In view of their amazing dexterity, it is not surprising that hands are very complex. Unfortunately, the hands, with their multitude of joints, are a major target of RA. Since the disease eventually affects the hands of all sufferers, let us examine them in some detail.

Bones and Joints

Each hand has 27 bones (see Fig. 13-1). The bones are subdivided into carpals that form the wrist, metacarpals that form the palm, and phalanges that form the digits (fingers). Strong ligaments connect the eight small, roundish carpal bones. The five metacarpals are elongated. Except for the thumb, which has only two, each finger consists of three elongated bones called phalanges (singular: phalanx). From the palm out, these phalanges are called:

- Proximal phalanges
- Middle phalanges
- Distal phalanges

To figure out which finger or joint is which, remember that in medicine the part closest to the center of the body is called *proximal* and the more distant part is called *distal*. Moreover, the little finger side of the hand is called the *ulnar* side, after the ulna (outside) bone of the arm. The thumb side of the hand is called the *radial* side, after the radius, the proximal bone of the arm. When physicians talk of ulnar drift, they mean that your fingers are leaning toward the little finger side of the hand. In

FIGURE 13-1. The Hand.

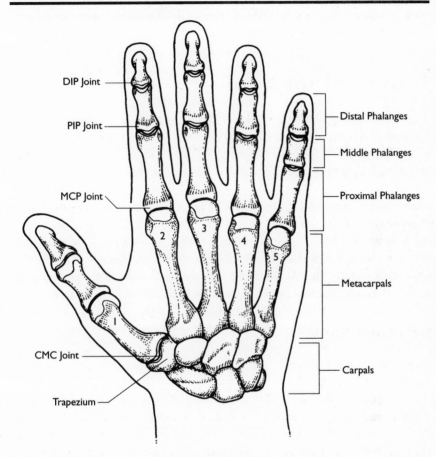

From The Columbia Presbyterian Osteoarthritis Handbook, *R. P. Grelsamer and S. Loebl, eds. Macmillan, 1996. Reproduced with permission.*

addition, health professionals dealing with the hand may talk of the *dorsal* side of the hand, which is the back of the hand, or the *volar* side, which is the palm side.

The joints of the hand are named after the bones they connect:

◆ Carpal-metacarpal joint (CMC)

◆ Metacarpal-phalangeal joint (MCP)

◆ Proximal interphalangeal joint (PIP)

◆ Distal interphalangeal joint (DIP)

All these joints are of the hinge type. The joint between the base of the thumb and the carpal bone, called the *trapezium,* is the trapeziometacarpal joint (TM). It swivels, providing the thumb with extra mobility.

In healthy joints there is adequate joint space between the bones of the fingers. Partial loss of this space (joint narrowing) is a sign of joint damage.

The bones of the hand form one longitudinal (lengthwise) arch and two transversal (crosswise) arches. These may collapse if RA damages the delicate architecture of the hand.

Muscles and Tendons

The muscles of the hand are divided into two groups: the extrinsic muscles (originating in the forearm) and the intrinsic muscles (originating in the hand itself). Both govern hand movement. The *extrinsic muscles* consist of long extensor and flexor muscles that provide power to the fingers and thumb. The *intrinsic muscles* govern the smaller movements required to execute fine balance and precision. Muscles as well as strong tendons (which attach muscles to bone) and ligaments (which attach bone to bone) keep the bones of the hand in place and maintain the overall architecture.

Nerves

Three major nerves—median, ulnar, and radial—innervate the hand. Information is transmitted by these nerves to and from the central nervous system (the brain and spinal cord). The space in the brain devoted to processing this information is large, again underlining the importance of the hands. All purposeful hand movements are initiated in the brain, and sensory input (e.g., pain, touch) from the fingers initiates immediate feedback.

THE HANDS AND RHEUMATOID ARTHRITIS

The inflammatory processes that affect the joints of the upper extremities do not differ markedly from those that occur elsewhere in the body. The initial symptom(s) is pain caused by the synovitis of the affected joint and possibly tendinitis (inflammation of the covering sheath of the tendon). An army of white blood cells invades the joint, a pannus forms, bones may erode, tendons and ligaments may weaken and even rupture, and nerves may become compressed.

Because finger joints are small and poorly protected by muscle tissue, these changes may rapidly affect the delicate architecture and function of the hand.

Common Hand Deformities

RA can twist the human hand into a multitude of shapes. The disease often affects one tendon more than another, thereby creating an imbalance in the structures that keep fingers properly aligned. In addition to the functional loss, these very obvious deformities carry with them a certain stigma. However, surgical intervention for cosmetic reasons alone is not recommended. Surgery is considered primary in those patients with limitation in hand function.

In advanced disease, the finger's three-joint system may collapse because tendons and ligaments lose their ability to prevent a particular joint from bending backward (hyperextension). The hyperextension or instability of one joint can in turn result in the flexion of the adjacent joint in the same finger. The most common hand abnormalities are as follows:

* *Swan-neck deformity:* This deformity usually involves two or three joints—for example, a fixed MIP and DIP joint and a hyperextended PIP joint. A swan-neck deformity interferes with grasping objects.

* *Boutonniere (buttonhole) deformity or mallet deformity:* The name of this deformity accurately describes the fact that the end of the finger drops.

* *Ulnar drift:* Even in health, the fingers may point toward the ulnar (outside) side of the hand. This tendency is magnified in RA. Fingers deviate at the MCP joints, sometimes making the hand look as if it is signaling.

Preventing Hand Deformities

As always, the first order of business is to prevent or limit deformity of the affected joints. For the hands the occupational therapist uses three different interrelated modalities:

1. Avoidance of any activity that puts excessive stress on the affected hand joints

2. Splinting the hand to prevent dislocations, decrease deformity, and or provide a correct resting position

3. Exercises

Protecting the Joints from Stress

These general suggestions were developed by the Hospital for Special Surgery's Department of Rehabilitation following the principles of joint protection and energy conservation:

1. When possible, use large joints to accomplish tasks: your wrist and palm, instead of your fingers; your elbow instead of your wrist; your shoulder rather than your elbow. Use two hands instead of one. Rely on various aids to independent living whenever you can.

2. Use shoulder straps on bags or briefcases. Avoid gripping the handles of your handbag with your fingers. Hang the handbag over the forearm instead.

3. Use two hands to hold a cup or a mug.

4. Do not grip a book when reading. Instead, prop a pillow across your knees or use it as a bookstand.

5. If you must use your fingers—for example, when using a keyboard at a computer or piano—rest and stretch your fingers and wrists every 10 to 15 minutes.

6. Never twist—or squeeze with—your fingers. Avoid wringing out a washcloth. Do not twist off bottle caps, peel oranges, pull on zippers, twist keys, or do the myriad of other tasks that combine force with finger dexterity. Use self-help devices instead.

7. Utilize levers to open doors.

Splinting

Our ancestors must have stabilized a broken or impaired limb with wooden sticks fastened with reeds. Splinting is the oldest effective orthopedic procedure. As in the past, splinting is used to stabilize an impaired joint. For those suffering from RA, splinting is used to rest, prevent, and even reverse arthritic deformities.

A sophisticated understanding of the functional anatomy of the hand has replaced guesswork, and the exact configuration of a splint is very precise. The goal of splints is usually to accomplish one or more of the following:

1. Immobilize a painful, inflamed joint

2. Prevent a joint from contracting by maintaining proper joint alignment

3. Prevent repetitive stress in a joint during activity

4. Improve joint function by increasing support and stability

5. Maintain surgical corrections

The physician or orthopedic surgeon prescribes the splint. The occupational therapist fabricates a customized splint, sees that it fits, and teaches the patient how to use it. Custom-made splints are made out of thermoplastic sheeting or neoprene that can be molded easily under hot water. Splints can also be ordered from catalogs. Velcro fastenings make it easy to take the splint on and off. Splints vary in complexity. Some are as simple as a soft collar, worn to stabilize the vertebrae of the neck. Others are as complex as the dynamic splints used after hand surgery.

Splints can be static, which means that they have no moving parts and maintain the joint in the desired position. Simple silver rings, which look like jewelry, are often used to stabilize finger joints.

Dynamic splints attempt to move the joint in a specific direction by exerting a dynamic force—for example, the complex splint worn after MP joint arthroplasty using silastic MP joint replacement (see Chapter 19) This splint puts an adjustable traction on individual fingers. Common problems requiring splinting and the splints used for correction are listed in Table 13-1. Splints are also used to relieve pressure on specific nerves (carpal tunnel syndrome.)

What to Ask About Your Splint

Useful as they are, splints are sometimes cumbersome to wear. It is thus extremely important that you discuss your splint with your therapist and ask what it will allow you to do. A splint is only useful when worn, and if wearing it is uncomfortable or limits your function, you should consult your therapist. The goal of the splint should be clearly outlined by your occupational therapist.

Compared to the drugs you take or the surgical procedures you may undergo, splints look rather harmless. A poorly fitting splint, however,

TABLE 13-1. Common Hand Problems and the Splints Used to Correct the Condition

Problem	Type of Splint	Desired Effect
Acute synovitis of the wrist	Volar wrist cock-up	Provides wrist support while allowing fingers to move.
Synovitis of the wrist and hand	Resting hand splint	Provides rest for wrist, MCP and IP joints, and thumb. Only worn at night.
Carpal tunnel syndrome	Volar or dorsal wrist support	Holds wrist in neutral position, thereby relieving pressure on median nerve. Usually only worn at night.
Ulnar drift at MCP joints	Volar splint with finger separators	Allows use of hand while preventing ulnar deviation.
Synovitis and teno-synovitis of various joints of the thumb	Various short thumb splints	Stabilize the wrist and restrict flexion of the affected joints of the thumb.
Swan-neck deformities	Figure of eight or silver ring splints	Apply three-point pressure to restrict hyperextension of the PIP joint. The splints allow flexion.

Adapted from "Occupational Therapy," by Toni Golin, in *Manual of Rheumatology and Outpatient Orthopedic Disorders*. Lippincott, Philadelphia, 1995.

may do more harm than good. Since splints may make the difference between a functional hand and one altered by disease, it is crucial that you have the answers to the following questions:

◆ What is the purpose of the splint?

◆ When and for how long should you wear the splint?

◆ Should you wear the splint when you bathe and shower?

◆ How do you put the splint on and take it off? (After washing your hands, make sure that the skin is dry before putting the splint back on.

- Should you do any hand exercises? Which ones?

- How you can tell if you have put the splint on correctly?

- What should you do if the skin under the splint becomes irritated?

- Watch out for pressure sores—i.e., redness that does not fade within 15 minutes. Call the therapist.

- Who should you call if you have trouble?

- What should you do if your arm, hand, or fingers feel numb, throb, or swell? (It is most likely that the splint is on too tight. Most splints fit correctly when you can put a finger under the strap. If the problem persists, remove the splint and call your therapist. If you have been instructed not to remove the splint, phone the therapist for instructions and/or an immediate appointment.)

How to Care for and Clean Your Splint

Thermoplastic may melt. It is important to keep your splint away from heat sources such as sunlight, hot water, and radiators.

Splints that are worn for prolonged periods of time need to be cleaned as follows:

- The stockinette that covers the hand splints can be washed in soap and water.

- To remove odors, apply a paste made from baking soda and water to the inner surface of the splint. Rinse with water and let dry.

- Replace broken rubber bands with the spares provided by your therapist.

EXERCISE

The Computer as an Exerciser

Annabel Griffith, an occupational therapist at the Hospital for Special Surgery, watches as Mrs. M. attempts to catch a series of bouncing red balls in a small bucket. The two are not in a gym—they're in front of a small computer screen! Annabel's enthusiasm for the manual upper limb exerciser (MULE) is obvious.

Traditionally, occupational therapists relied on arts and crafts. Patients wove potholders, made collages, and performed other tasks to exercise and rehabilitate their hands. Ten years ago, occupational therapists in England developed computer software and a series of tool attachments that allow patients to exercise their hands, wrists, forearms, elbows, and shoulders.

The exerciser comes with eight different attachments designed so that the patients use different grips and pinching motions to play nine different computer games designed to increase or maintain motion, grip and pinch strength, and fine motor coordination. The games also require good eye-hand coordination, concentration, and many other complex processes that make the human hand such an amazing tool.

In the Balls and Bucket game, the player moves the bucket across the lower edge of the screen by rotating one of the tool attachments. The therapist varies the difficulty of this game by adjusting the number of balls and the speed at which they fall. The bucket can also be moved across the screen by means of any hand attachment chosen. The machine does not isolate one particular joint, but enables the patient to exercise all the joints required for normal hand use.

The MULE scores a patient's performance. As patients improve, their score rises. This provides tremendous encouragement and a sense of achievement, thereby increasing the patient's self-confidence and enthusiasm for rehabilitation.

Traditional Exercises

As for other joints, a hand therapist carefully prescribes exercises. The movements of a healthy hand are closely related to other joints of the arm. Depending on the status of the disease, exercises may be contraindicated. During the inflammatory phase, there are no exercises, and therapy focuses on correct immobilization and edema control. It is important to follow the instructions provided by the therapist. For instance, when instructed to exercise, patients should not alter the prescription—that is, the number of repetitions—without speaking to the therapist.

In general, active range of motion exercises (performed without assistance) aim to maintain, restore, and only sometimes increase motion. Passive range of motion exercises (performed with additional force provided by the therapist or patient) are sometimes contraindicated because RA joints are unstable.

Patients are encouraged to use their hands for functional tasks as opposed to wearing out their joints with unnecessary exercises. A limited exercise program is valuable to prevent morning stiffness and maintain motion in all joints of the upper extremities. These exercises should be carefully prescribed.

Pain Relief

Hands are meant to be extremely sensitive, and an inflamed finger joint can hurt a lot. In addition to the usual pain-relief medications, many patients love a paraffin bath. Molten (warm, not hot) paraffin coats the hand like a glove and slowly gives off heat as it cools. Inserting the paraffin-coated hand into a plastic bag can delay the cooling.

Small paraffin baths for home use cost about $140. (One source is Grimm, P.O. Box 2143, Marietta, OH 45750; 800-223-5395.) Medicare and/or other insurance usually reimburse the cost. Such baths can also be bought at department stores.

Since the finger joints are close to the surface, relief can sometimes be obtained through the application of topical analgesic creams.

Problem Solving

The assessment questionnaire discussed at the beginning of this chapter will give you and the occupational therapist a pretty good idea of what you can and cannot do. Together you will solve some of your immediate problems. You will solve others on your own as time goes on. Here are some general suggestions. Again, the advice only scratches the surface:

1. Living with any chronic disease unfortunately requires patience. Everything will take longer than it did before you became ill.

2. *An ounce of prevention is worth a pound of cure* applies to RA. Protect your affected joints. If the arthritis affects your weight-bearing joints, avoid standing while you work in the kitchen. Use assistance devices if the arthritis affects your hands.

3. Order the book *Guide to Independent Living for People with Arthritis* from the Arthritis Foundation. The book is full of suggestions on how to do most things. It includes advice on toileting, meal preparation, sewing, gardening, cutting up your meat, taking care of your baby, and much, much more. Many of the suggestions are very simple—for example, a rubber mat keeps plates and bowls from slipping.

Large knobs help you turn lights on and off. Long-handled brooms and dustpans relieve some of the stress related to keeping house.

4. It is usually best to solve problems permanently—for example, if it is difficult for you to turn a key, acquire a key holder. Cover your doorknobs with a lever to avoid stressing the wrist. Ask your pharmacist to provide easy-to-open medicine bottles.

5. Organize your tasks. For an active person used to doing the laundry while cooking dinner, or planning dinner at the last moment and rushing all over the place to locate ingredients, this adjustment is difficult. In the end, however, having whatever you need in one place—recipes, spices, chopping board, pans, special knives—will save a lot of wear and tear.

6. Overcome your reluctance and ask for help. If this is emotionally difficult, imagine how you would feel if the shoe were on the other foot. Chances are that you would gladly help a friend in need.

7. Learn how to use a computer. This not only avoids or decreases the strain of writing with pencil and paper, but also allows you to share in what is going on in the world. The Internet enables you to socialize at home. There are many chat rooms for people sharing interests, and you can even play bridge or chess. Ask your therapist about the position of your hands while typing. Make sure that your hands are straight and not bent at the wrist for any length of time.

8. Do not waste strength on shopping. Make a list and either call a store that delivers or have members of your family do the grocery shopping. Shop from catalogs for clothes and gifts. Use the Internet to order books, appliances, and supplies.

9. Avoid lifting. While cooking, slide pots onto the stove. Transport books, briefcases, and other stuff in a small shopping cart or strapped to wheels.

10. Traveling with RA takes planning. Take advantage of the conveniences offered by airlines and bus companies. Order a wheelchair when traveling by plane and ask the bus driver to lower the step so that you can get on and off the bus.

11. When cooking and eating, use your healthier joints.

14

Coping with Rheumatoid Arthritis

———————≈«◎»≈———————

This chapter offers suggestions on how to deal with pain, depression, and other physical and emotional problems associated with a disease whose manifestations are unpredictable. Some of the suggestions are derived from patients attending an education program at the Hospital for Special Surgery.

Helen looked at the clock: 3 A.M.! How could a little finger hurt that much? Should she get up and get an ice pack? A hot pack? Make a cup of tea? Get that no-good cream that was supposed to temporarily relieve the pain of arthritis? She was too exhausted to do any of that, so she just stayed in bed and massaged the small, warm joint. She knew that within days or weeks the pain in her pinkie would subside, but then it would be the turn of another joint or joints. Last month it was her knees, and before that it was one of her thumbs.

Pain has a purpose. It protects the body from injury. "Ouch," your mind screams when you touch a hot stove. Before you realize it, you have withdrawn your hand. In RA, however, pain is out of control, it is constant, and it requires special attention. The pain you experience has many different causes: damaged joints, inflammation, tense muscles, emotional losses.

PAIN THRESHOLD

In *The Columbia Presbyterian Osteoarthritis Handbook,* the authors recall Hans Christian Andersen's tale of *The Princess and the Pea.* One night, a princess visits the castle of an eligible bachelor prince. Mindful of a possible impersonator, the mother of the prince hides a pea in the guest bed concealed by one hundred mattresses. The next morning, when asked how she had slept, the girl replied that she had slept very poorly and that her body was "black and blue." The queen was satisfied, for "only a true princess would have been sensitive enough to be bothered by a pea cushioned by one hundred mattresses."

Real people also have very different pain thresholds. During your treatment you will be asked repeatedly to grade your pain from zero or one to ten, zero being no pain, ten being maximum. Your own pain threshold varies from day to day, week to week, and month to month. When your disease is in remission, you may be able to tolerate quite a bit of discomfort. When the disease acts up, you may sympathize with the princess and her pea. Many factors play a role in pain perception: anxiety, depression, the weather, anticipation of discomfort, sleep deprivation and fatigue, to name only a few.

A person's response to pain relief measures is also highly individual. A minor painkiller will do wonders for some; others hurt in spite of high doses of more powerful medication. Some people love acupuncture; others respond to massage, imagery, heat, or cold. In time, you will discover the measures that help you the most.

Pain is not always the same. There is a vast difference between dull, aching morning stiffness, the acute pain of a joint that refuses to work properly, and the burning sensation of inflamed tissue. And there is not only physical pain. Even the best patient occasionally becomes discouraged and depressed.

TRADITIONAL METHODS OF PAIN CONTROL

Drug Therapy

The alleviation of pain is medicine's oldest preoccupation. Our ancestors discovered the opiates. Alcohol was used to dull pain during surgery before the discovery of anesthetics, and mild painkillers such as aspirin and acetaminophen have been available for over a century. Today, physicians have dozens of additional pain-relieving medications (see Chapter 7). Taking these drugs as needed is an important aspect of your self-care. Remember that pain begets pain. It is best to keep pain under control. Take your medication before you embark on a stressful physical or mental activity.

There is much more than medication to pain relief. This chapter deals with nonpharmacological aspects of this crucial subject.

Physical Measures

Heat

One of the best ways of relieving joint pain is through the application of heat:

- It decreases joint stiffness.

- It lessens pain.

- It relieves muscle spasms.

- It increases blood flow.

Heat improves vasodilation (increases diameter of blood vessels) and thus the healing effects of blood flow. Therapeutically, heat application is subdivided into superficial heat and deep heat.

Superficial heat, as provided by a soothing, warm bath or hot shower, an electric blanket, or a mattress pad, does wonders. To minimize morning stiffness, turn the heat of these appliances up for 20 minutes before you get out of bed.

Hot water bottles, various compresses, and electric heating pads provide localized, dry heat. (Be careful to turn these off before you go to sleep and avoid using these gadgets on freshly operated wounds or damaged skin.)

For poorly understood reasons, moist heat is more effective than dry heat. A towel soaked in warm water, or a damp towel heated in the microwave, makes a simple compress. Your local drugstore or various mail-order companies can supply you with a variety of ElastoGel hot/cold wraps adapted to various parts of the body. Buying some of these is a wise investment. Paraffin baths (see Chapter 13) provide relief for painful hands and feet. Therapists recommend applying heat for 20 to 30 minutes at a time, though this is different for each patient.

A physical therapist or other trained professional usually administers deep heat treatments, in which heat is delivered directly to the underlying affected area. During these modalities, one type of energy—

most often diathermy (using short waves) or ultrasound (high-energy sound waves)—is transformed into deep heat. During both procedures, the energy source is applied to the region of the body closest to the involved joint.

Diathermy, which mobilizes joints and decreases pain, is not indicated for patients with metallic surgical implants because the radiation concentrates in metal. Metal jewelry and clothing with metallic fasteners must be removed before the initiation of this therapy.

Ultrasound therapy is much like diathermy. It, too, improves joint function, mobilizes frozen joints, relieves muscle tension, and may be beneficial for the overall health of connective tissue. It should be used cautiously in patients with total joint replacement because the high-energy waves may possibly weaken the methylmethacrylate glue used to anchor the prosthesis.

Cold

Cold, which initially causes a numbing effect, is commonly and effectively used to relieve the pain of acutely inflamed, injured, and newly operated-on joints. Initially, cold causes vasoconstriction (narrowing of the blood vessels), thereby decreasing the flow of inflammation mediators from the site of injury to the central nervous system. Eventually, vasoconstriction is followed by vasodilation and a beneficial improved blood flow. To make a cold compress, use an ice bag, ice cubes wrapped in a towel, a bag of frozen peas, or commercially available ElastoGel packs.

Transcutaneous Electric Nerve Stimulation (TENS)

This method involves the delivery of low-intensity electric impulses to the affected area. During the procedure, a therapist tapes electrodes to the skin near the treated joint. The delivery of a varying intensity current to the joint is accompanied by a low-grade tingling sensation. Nobody knows why TENS provides pain relief in some patients. Some practitioners believe that the procedure releases endorphins, the body's own opiates, whereas others think that TENS overloads the nerve paths, thereby overriding the pain impulses.

Immobilization and Joint Protection

Keeping an injured, painful limb from moving is instinctive. Splinting inflamed joints may relieve pain, prevent or limit deformity, and stabilize the joint. Professionally made splints are an important aspect of therapy. Splints must be used strictly under medical supervision because they immobilize the muscles tissue surrounding a joint and promote muscle atrophy. Chapter 13 provides detailed information on splints.

ALTERNATIVE METHODS OF PAIN CONTROL
Massage

Most everybody enjoys getting a massage. Because massages release stress, relax tense muscles, improve blood flow, and alleviate pain, they are especially soothing for people suffering from musculoskeletal disorders. Until a few decades ago, massages were looked at askance because masseuses were sometimes used as a cover for prostitution. Today, massages have gone mainstream. The 29,000 registered practitioners are certified by the American Massage Therapy Association (AMTA). Sometimes—though rarely—massages are reimbursed by medical insurance. (For reimbursement purposes, massage therapy should be prescribed by a physician, and, if possible, should be coupled with an exercise program.)

There is something ritualistic about a good massage. Clients are welcomed into a pleasant, sometimes scented room. They may undress, don a sheet or gown, and lie on a massage table. They may be asked what part of the body hurts most. The therapist applies a few drops of oil and may turn on some music.

The 80 or so forms of massage therapy differ from one another mostly in the type of stroke used and in the depth of the tissues reached by the therapist. Swedish massage is the most widely used technique. It consists of long, even strokes and gentle kneading, both of which relieve muscle spasms, lessen pain, and improve blood circulation. Some forms of massage, such as Rolfing, go much deeper. Therapists use their knuckles, thumbs, and fingers to relieve stress in specific muscle groups. Massage therapists take great pride in their work and no two massages are exactly alike.

You may wince as the masseur or masseuse kneads and presses on the many sore spots of your body. You may be surprised to discover in how many different places you can hurt. But it is a good hurt, which is followed by a wonderful feeling of being freed from pain, if only for a very short time.

Massages are not curative, and their beneficial effect is poorly understood. A good therapist, however, can do wonders for people in pain.

RA patients should select a massage therapist who is familiar with the disease.

The AMTA has a Web site at: www.amtamassage.org. Its *Find a Massage Therapist* locator service, listing their membership, can be reached at 847–864–0123.

Acupressure is a variant in which the masseur or masseuse concentrates on applying presses to the acupuncture points.

Acupuncture

Ever since it arrived in the West during the 1970s, acupuncture has puzzled the medical establishment. Chinese physicians have used the procedure for more than 2,500 years to relieve pain. It is so effective that in China it is sometimes used instead of anesthesia for major surgical procedures. Numerous experiments have attempted to understand the physiological basis of acupuncture.

Scientists have confirmed that the insertion of needles into traditional acupuncture points can cause multiple biological responses resulting in the activation of pathways affecting various physiological systems in the brain as well as in the periphery. This triggers the release of the endorphins (endogenous opioids) that are responsible for the analgesia. (From NIH Consensus Statement, 1997). Acupuncture alters the flow of neurotransmitters, immune function, and regulation of blood flow. None of these effects, however, are long-lasting. The procedure seems to be most effective for postoperative pain and for the relief of nausea and vomiting associated with chemotherapy and perhaps pregnancy. Its effect in RA is unclear. Not everybody responds to acupuncture. The percentage of responders is unknown.

Biofeedback

In this method, successfully used to alter certain physiological pathways, patients train their minds to relax certain muscle groups. In a typical setup, the patient is sitting in a small, soundproof, dimly lit booth, with electrodes taped to the head. The electrodes record an electric potential related to muscle tension. Additional instruments convert this tension to a feedback signal such as a click. The tenser the muscles, the faster the click. Gradually, the patient learns what thoughts and sensations increase or decrease the speed of the signal. The patient gradually learns to relax the muscles without being tethered to the machine.

For more information on nondrug methods of pain control, see also Judith Horstman, *The Arthritis Foundation's Guide to Alternative Therapies* (Arthritis Foundation, Atlanta, Georgia, 1999).

LIFESTYLE CHANGES

For years, Doris suffered from pain, in her case caused by a debilitating back. Then, one day, mostly because her ungainly shape disgusted her, she signed up for an exercise class. Gradually her dependence on pain medication decreased. She became stronger and happier and eventually was almost entirely pain-free.

Most patients with RA won't be that lucky, but exercise is a very successful method of pain control. Start the day by stretching in bed for at least 5 minutes. Chances are that your morning stiffness will decrease in time and perhaps also in intensity. For details on exercise and RA, see Chapter 12.

MIND OVER MATTER

Every so often, the Patient Education Department of HSS organizes a self-help group for patients suffering from RA. Today, when such groups exist for every conceivable disease, it is interesting to recall that Dr. Joseph Hershey Pratt founded the first group in Boston in 1905. Pratt was in charge of tuberculosis (TB) patients at Massachusetts General Hospital. One of the acceptable treatments for TB in these preantibiotic days was fresh, crisp mountain air, but not every patient could afford this, and many had to remain in the slums of the rapidly expanding cities. Dr. Pratt organized "A Class for the Treatment of TB in the Homes of the Poor." At the regular meetings, patients shared experiences on how they managed to get as much fresh city air as possible. One patient slept on a fire escape; another pitched a tent on a roof. To everybody's surprise, Pratt's patients did as well or better than those who went to fancy mountain resorts. The therapeutic effect of a common bond in a common disease had been discovered.

This is the fourth meeting of the group organized by Adina Batterman, MSW. Once a month, about 20 people assemble on the seventh floor of the hospital. A look around the room indicates that rheumatoid arthritis does not discriminate. There are men and women (more women than men). The participants are a variety of ages and races. Even a casual observer notices swan necks, mallets, and other deformities, and some people have trouble picking up their sandwiches.

A feeling of confidence nevertheless prevails. These are mostly veterans who have accepted that they must deal with a painful, chronic disease. Even though they meet infrequently, the members of the group have already bonded. During the next 2 hours, they will share their frustrations and victories. "Nobody else can understand what this disease is like," says Jeanette D., who was diagnosed 3 years ago. "I am tired of people telling me that I look well and that my disease could not possibly be that bad."

Until now, the formal lectures dealt with safe subjects such as diet, exercise, and drugs. Today's talk on "How to Deal with the Stress of RA" is more personal. For patients suffering from RA, excess stress often translates into increased muscle tension and pain. There is even some evidence that stress may impact on the immune system. Stress also increases frustration, anger, hopelessness, and all the other negative feelings confronted by RA patients.

After a few introductory remarks, Roberta Horton, a social worker at HSS, asks the group what aspect of RA they find most stressful. The answers keep coming:

- Accepting the disease
- Parenting
- The unpredictability of RA
- The limitation of the body
- Dealing with depression
- Frustration of not being able to do the things once taken for granted
- Fear of the unknown
- Being afraid of not being able to care for oneself
- Becoming sharp and impatient with others
- The appearance of one's hands
- Pain, fatigue, and endless visits to doctors
- Taking medications that don't work

Unrehearsed, the group had enumerated the seven stressors that Patricia P. Katz identified in a large study of patients suffering from RA published in *Arthritis Care and Research* in February 1998. Katz's list is as follows:

1. Pain

2. Fatigue

3. Changes in joint appearance

4. Unpredictability of symptoms

5. Burden of taking care of RA

6. Functional impairment

7. Medication side effects

STRESS

To survive, all creatures are equipped to respond to danger. Even before we are totally aware of a threat, our body produces hormones that allow it to put up a good fight or flee to a safe harbor. To perform these increased demands, the extra hormones speed up the heart and respiratory rate, increase blood pressure, and tense the muscles. This preparedness also enables us to face other challenges such as sprinting at the end of a race, asking the boss for a raise, or giving a speech. Once the challenge is over, body function returns to normal.

Not all the stresses we encounter in life are good. Most people are stressed by rush-hour traffic, crowded beaches, and financial worries. Most everybody we know reports being stressed out. Their bodies may confirm their diagnosis by developing a tension headache or a knotted stomach.

RELAXATION AND STRESS RELIEF

Since pain headed the stressor list of this particular group, its relief was the first discussion topic. Pain, whether caused by an inflamed joint or an injury, is always in the head. It should not come as a surprise that the mind can play an important role in pain relief. Relaxation techniques are very effective in relieving stress and chronic pain.

The principle governing all relaxation techniques involves (temporarily) leaving the here and now and taking your mind elsewhere. You need to make yourself as comfortable as possible and breathe deeply, in and out, holding the breath while your lungs are full. Thereafter, techniques vary. You may be asked to visualize a peaceful setting, to recall your childhood home, or to repeat a mantra. You are instructed to relax your muscles or a group of muscles. It takes practice, but if relaxation works for you, stress and pain will subside.

Closely related to relaxation is visualization, first popularized in cancer therapy. The technique involves looking at the diseased portion of your body, such as an inflamed joint, confronting it in all its ugliness, and shrinking it to manageable proportions.

If relaxation and visualization work for you, you may wish to buy one or more of the audiotapes available at book and record stores, from catalogs, or from the Arthritis Foundation.

During her presentation at HSS, Roberta Horton suggested several quickie visualization exercises. The group liked the following adapted from *Wellness: An Arthritis Reality,* by Beth Zeibell:

> *Imagine a light bulb—just a plain old ordinary light bulb. Now move it slowly to the area of your pain. Turn on the light and allow the warmth to bring comfort. And now let the pain become the light—lower and lower until there is nothing left but a pleasant feeling of warmness.*

Many people in the group enjoyed the exercise. The mood lightened and one participant told a doctor's joke: "How many doctors does it take to change a light bulb?" Everyone laughed when they heard the answer. "It depends on what insurance you have."

Humor

It was Norman Cousins, one of America's leading writers, who discovered the healing power of laughter. Cousins was deathly sick with a form of inflammatory arthritis when he decided to "laugh himself well." Cousins retells his experience in his book, *Anatomy of an Illness* (W. W. Norton, 1991). After a hospital stay, Cousins, with the agreement of his physician, checked himself into a motel. His luggage included a bunch of goofy films including reels of *Candid Camera* and episodes of the Marx Brothers. Cousins watched the films and laughed—hearty belly laughs. Within a week, he felt better. Laughter, it appears, stimulates the immune system. By relaxing the muscles, changing our breathing pattern, and increasing blood circulation, it provides a wonderful physical workout. Humor also takes your mind off your pain and defuses tense family situations.

Getting to laugh is not always easy. Moreover, different things amuse different people. One person may love slapstick; another, political jokes; a third, cartoons. The Internet provides jokes (www.wizvax.net/humor), and you may buy one of several books that make you laugh. Best of all, you may know someone with whom you can share laughter.

Prayer

One day, when her son was facing a serious illness, Madeline unexpectedly wandered into a church. It happened to be a very wonderful church. Light was streaming through stained-glass windows. The organ was playing and the incantations of the priest were soothing. For the first time in weeks, peace was enveloping Madeline's mind. Even though she was not a believer, Madeline kept returning to services. The stillness of the sanctuary and the realization that none of the other worshippers knew of her heartache were healing. Madeline left the church strengthened, ready once more to face her heavy burden. For some people, formal or informal prayer may be a wonderful way of relieving stress and pain.

GRIEF AND RA (WHY ME?)

It takes a while, even for the best adjusted among us, to accept that we are suffering from a lifelong chronic disease. When serious illness strikes, we are incredulous, and before we are willing and able to deal with this reality, we must mourn our former, healthy selves. Such grieving progresses via several well-defined stages: denial, anger, bargaining, depression, and finally acceptance.

There is no way of predicting of how many months or years each stage will take, and nobody is ever done with the grief cycle once and for all. People who have made peace with a major loss find that at unexpected times it again becomes acute, to be dealt with all over again. Some people may be incapable of ever completing the cycle.

Denial

Denial used to receive bad press. Today, it is considered to be a coping strategy that permits people to gradually accept a new reality. During denial people try to escape reality. Common thoughts are: The tests must be wrong. Or: I simply won't pay any attention to my pain. Or: I'll be able to lick this RA. Some people ignore the disease and go on with their lives as if there were no disease. Others become thoroughly depressed and isolated. Some rely entirely on unproven remedies. Most people go back and forth between overactivity and listlessness. Eventually, when the symptoms don't vanish, they become angry.

Anger

Anger never feels good. One patient of the HSS support group related how incensed she was when her fingers could not open a "stupid" bottle of water. "I was going to get that bottle open no matter what it took," she said. Others recalled how they got angry at everything and everybody, including their families. Anger does have its place in life and can be used successfully. Somebody recalled marching into the doctor's office and demanding better pain-relief medication. Others reported successful struggles with insurance companies. Eventually, most everyone feels guilty about being so angry and proceeds to the next stages.

Bargaining and Depression

When the reality of the disease sets in, people become depressed. They report being overwhelmed by fear, anxiety, and financial worries. This is the "Why me?" stage of the grieving process. You may doubt everything you, your doctor, your spouse, or your children say or do. Some people try to bargain. One person with RA recalls promising, "God, I will go to mass every day if you only stop my knee from hurting."

Acceptance

Eventually, most everyone is ready to deal with the here and now, and the sun sometimes peeks out from behind the clouds. "You have to rebuild your life," says Kathleen Lewis, RN, author and fellow sufferer. "You have to reinvent yourself. You'll become a different, perhaps better, person than you were." But Ms. Lewis cautions her audience that chronic disease is always a balancing act. Living with disease is living one day at a time. "Listen to yourself," she advises, "and do not minimize denial, depression, anger, or any other feelings that you may experience" (K. S. Lewis: *Successful Living with Chronic Illness,* Kendell Hunt, Dubuque, Iowa).

Even before you have made peace with RA, you have no choice but to go on with your life. You will have begun to cope. Most everyone is adamant about not wanting to be labeled a victim. This is why many arthritis sufferers become experts at self-management.

Having RA is difficult for both you and your family. A husband may have to spend more time taking care of the home and less time at his job or on the golf course. A wife may not be able to have a career. Your illness will consume some of the family's income. Remember that having RA is not your fault. You still are the person you were before you had RA.

INSOMNIA

Sleeping poorly is not restricted to people suffering from RA. According to the National Sleep Foundation, 70 million Americans—a third of the adult population—suffer from sleep problems. Sleeping poorly is a major symptom of fibromyalgia—a major form of arthritis—and is a problem for those suffering from RA.

Lack of sleep magnifies most aspects of RA. It increases pain and depression. Your muscles hurt more because they did not have a chance to relax. Your productivity decreases and it takes you longer to get things done. Table 14-1 offers suggestions on how to maximize your chances of having a good night's sleep. See also Suzanne Loebl's article "Counting on Sleep" in *Arthritis Today* (July/August 1998).

Chose a good, firm mattress. Make yourself as comfortable as you can, but the most comfortable position is not necessarily the healthiest as far as your joints are concerned. When an inflamed joint is kept in a bent position during the night, it may develop flexion contractures. Discuss your sleeping position with your physician, occupational therapist, or physical therapist. In general, to maintain neck alignment, support the neck with a small pillow or wear a soft collar. If you sleep on your side, a small pillow between your legs may alleviate stress on the hips and lower back. Sleeping on your back is best if you have hip and/or knee problems.

These recommendations do not mean that you must stay in one position. Moving around in your sleep keeps your joints from jelling and minimizes morning stiffness.

FATIGUE

It used to take Allison 30 minutes to prepare dinner. It was almost effortless. Now, even though she has simplified the menu, she finds making dinner exhausting. It is the same with housework.

TABLE 14-1. How to Promote Sleep

- Use your bedroom only for sleeping and sex.
- Always go to bed and get up at the same time.
- Try cutting out daytime naps.
- If pain interferes with your sleep, plan your medication so that it is effective during the nighttime.
- When you lie down, make yourself as comfortable as you can. Plan a quiet relaxing time before going to bed. Listen to soothing music or read a book.
- Take a warm bath before you go to sleep.
- Milk contains large amounts of tryptophan, an amino acid that promotes sleep. A glass of milk is a time-honored recipe for going to sleep.
- Avoid foods or beverages containing caffeine.
- Avoid alcohol for 3 to 4 hours before bedtime.
- Drink a cup of herb tea. Read the label to make sure it does not contain caffeine.
- Avoid strenuous exercise after 3:00 P.M. Languorous stretches, on the other hand, promote sleep.
- Avoid eating heavy meals close to bedtime. Do not overload your body with fluids.
- If you have trouble falling asleep, use one of your relaxation exercises. Visit your childhood home, imagine yourself on vacation, or count sheep.
- If you do wake up and can't go back to sleep within 20 minutes, get up and repeat your evening routine. Stay up until you are sleepy.

High on the list of the miseries associated with RA is fatigue. "I feel as if I had the flu," says one patient. "I just don't want to get up in the morning and start," says another. "I am always tired," says a third.

Fatigue is really an ill-defined symptom caused by the physical burden of the disease. Sometimes it may be due to anemia, which often accompanies RA. Trying to do things while fatigued only makes matters worse. Chances are you'll become ill humored and depressed.

Admitting to yourself that RA is forcing you to give up many of the things you used to do effortlessly is perhaps the hardest adjustment to make. The following suggestions may help you feel you are getting your jobs done and remaining in control:

- Identify what events (excess work, no rest, standing, late nights) trigger more than average fatigue and try to eliminate them.

- Prioritize, plan, and delegate.

- Become an expert list maker for organizing your day.

- Decrease your overall workload.

- Arrange your activities in such a way that you alternate physically taxing ones such as vacuuming or gardening with restful ones such as sewing, filing, or sitting at the computer.

- Minimize needlessly taxing activities such as shopping in an over-crowded supermarket.

- Be flexible. Always have frozen food in reserve for when you are tired.

DEPRESSION

The alarm clock rang. It was Tuesday, and Ernest was supposed to get ready for his exercise class. But he could not get out of bed. "The exercises won't help me anyhow," he thought. Finally, Ernest got up. He missed half the class, and when he came back home, he was exhausted. He went back to bed and slept some more. The phone rang. He did not answer it but turned on the TV instead. That did not help. War was raging in Eastern Europe, the stock market fell, the ozone level was high... Ernest was depressed.

Erica was depressed, too. She had a date with friends to go shopping in the new mall, but before she even got out of bed she knew that this was going to be a bad day. Since she had been diagnosed with RA 3 years ago, nothing ever went right. Reluctantly, she got up, did a few stretches, and made some coffee. After a while, she felt better. Then she had a thought: Perhaps she could join her friends for lunch.

Many people suffering from RA are depressed some of the time. But there is a vast difference between Ernest and Erica. Chronic illness is governed by a complex interplay between mood and disease. This is especially marked in RA, whose direct manifestations and consequences elicit depression. Common triggers are:

- Pain and fatigue

- Emotional isolation

- Giving up many pleasurable activities

- Having to spend so much time taking care of one's body

- Side effects of medications

- Loss of control
- Fear of the future

Depression is a major health problem, not necessarily related to RA. It has plagued humankind since antiquity. It is of interest that Robert Burton, a dean of Oxford University, wrote *The Anatomy of Melancholy* in 1621, which describes the symptoms of his own depression.

What Can Be Done About Depression?

The treatment of depression depends on its intensity. Ernest's paralyzing depression needs prompt medical attention. Erica will probably be able to manage on her own. The extent of your depression depends in part on your personality and your outlook on life.

Here are a few suggestions on how to handle depression. Some of the interventions will sound familiar. Some remedies, such as exercise and positive thought processes, are so useful that they lift depression, decrease stress, and mitigate pain:

- Recognize depression and examine its causes. If it is severe, all-inclusive, and accompanied by suicidal thoughts, consult your physician immediately. If you feel that you can cope on your own, try to analyze the cause of your depression. Accept sadness.

- Talk to your doctor or therapist about your feelings. You may profit from a change in medication or even some mood-elevating medication such as Prozac.

- Join a support group or find a phone buddy. The Internet even provides chat rooms for people suffering from chronic disease.

- Keep a diary. Recent research has proven that keeping a diary about one's pain, moods, and other events is very helpful. Record keeping imposes some order on seeming chaos. The Serenity Prayer, used by many 12-step programs (give me the strength to change what can be changed, accept what cannot be changed, and the wisdom to know the difference) is powerful because it applies to so many situations.

- Figure out what triggers your depression—for example, being treated as an invalid, having unrelenting pain, having to forego specific pleasures, being suspected of being lazy. Attempt to defuse the situations that bother you the most.

- Exercise for 30 minutes a day.

- Develop new favorite activities to substitute for those that no longer fit. Giving up a favorite activity is painful; however, substituting a treadmill or an exercise bike for aerobics or walking for jogging may work. In time, most everybody accepts the fact that his or her physical ability and endurance are limited. It is also important to listen to your body and avoid overexertion.

- Look your best. Put on nice clothes every day, style your hair, put on makeup, shave, and so forth, even when you stay home alone. You'll feel better when you look at yourself in the mirror.

COGNITIVE THERAPY

Every so often, somebody invents a new mousetrap, and sometimes, indeed, it is better. A couple of decades ago, David D. Burns, M.D., and his associates at the University of Pennsylvania Medical Center, developed a new approach to defusing attitudes that are particularly damaging to people suffering from chronic diseases. This so-called mood therapy is based on cognitive thinking. *Cognate* refers to knowing and understanding. Dr. Burns demonstrated that negative thoughts are detrimental and often result in depression. In addition, negative thoughts are frequently distorted—for example: "My car does not start. I will have to junk it." By analyzing and challenging such unrealistic thought processes, people can prevent feeling hopeless.

Burns lists 10 principal cognitive distortions. At the HSS support meeting, Roberta Horton discussed the list. Here are examples of how distortions might affect people suffering from RA:

1. *All-or-nothing thinking:* "This new medication does not work. There is no medication that works for my kind of RA."

2. *Overgeneralization:* "My boss does not understand that my RA really makes me feel tired. He thinks that I am lazy. Everybody thinks that I am goofing off."

3. *Mental filter:* Mary expected her friend, Robert, to call her on Tuesday. When he did not call, she was convinced that he would never call again, ignoring the fact that Robert had driven her to school that morning.

4. *Disqualifying the positive:* Arthur complimented Betsy on her new haircut. Betsy thought of her twisted hands and was convinced that Arthur was just being nice to make her feel good.

5. *Jumping to conclusions:* Philip, a real estate broker, sold an expensive house. At a staff meeting, the head of the company failed to compliment him on the sale. Philip concluded that his boss felt that he should have made additional sales.

6. *Magnification (or minimization):* You magnify your shortcomings—for example: "I cannot go on class trips with my son. I am a bad mother." Or: "All my daughter's friends love to come to my house after school, but that is unimportant."

7. *Emotional reasoning:* "I feel like a failure, so I must be a failure."

8. *Should statements:* Your RA flares. You blame yourself because you should have exercised more.

9. *Labeling and mislabeling:* You and 10 other people apply for a job. You do not get the job and tell yourself that you are a born loser.

10. *Personalization:* You assume that everything bad that happens to you or your family is your fault. Your mother breaks a leg and you think that it is your fault because you should have made sure that she got rid of the scatter rug in the front hall.

Roberta Horton illustrated how such distortions can be diffused so as to forestall activating a negative chain reaction. Ms. Horton used Burns's four-column technique to challenge the inability of carrying out plans, a situation often encountered by people suffering from RA (for additional details, see *Feeling Good,* by David D. Burns, Morrow, 1980):

Activating Event	Automatic Thought	Cognitive Distortion	Realistic Reappraisal
It is hot, 97°, and very humid. I have to cancel my plans.	I'll never leave the house all summer.	Overgeneralization, magnification, jumping to conclusions	I am really disappointed. I'll try for the movies at night.

SEX

"If I were Bob, I would hate me," Shirley T. was telling her Florida neighbor. "Last year, I had two flares and was miserable. This year, everything was fine, but then I cracked three ribs. That hurt so much that I screamed whenever I got dressed. And then my ulcer started to act up. Fortunately, I nipped that crisis in the bud." Bob, of course, had no intention of divorcing his wife. As a matter of fact, most of their friends envy the T's loving relationship even though Shirley developed RA 25 years ago. Eventually, she also developed ulcers and osteoporosis, both a result of long-term corticosteroid therapy. Even though Bob feels sorry for Shirley, he does not treat her as an invalid. Together they've taken many trips, raised a son, and are now close to their two grandchildren.

Serious illness interferes with carefree relationships including sex. Even though sex is no longer as taboo a subject as it used to be, most everybody has trouble talking about it, especially when external factors, such as a serious illness, intrude. Dissatisfaction with your sex life, however, does not necessarily start with RA. Chances are that if it was good and solid, it can continue to be so. If it was rocky, RA won't help.

As with most other aspects of the disease, sexual issues can be subdivided into physiological and psychological problems. Pain and fatigue obviously are sexual downers. Handle these as best as you can by planning your sexual activities for when you are least tired and your pain medication is maximally effective. A hot bath that relaxes your joints may also help. Depending on the composition of your household, such planning may not work. If feasible, you may plan for a weekend away from home. A mini-vacation may do wonders for your relationship, regardless of whether you actually have intercourse.

Painful, inflamed joints and depression, which often accompany RA, interfere with sex. Information on sexual positions that protect painful joints is readily available. Trial and error may help you discover satisfying positions. Vaginal dryness, which is a problem for many women, is often relieved by appropriate external lubrication. Be aware that certain medications, especially tranquilizers and antidepressants, often decrease libido.

Psychological problems interfering with sex may yield to improved communication. Talking dispels misconceptions and clarifies what each partner wants from the other. You may wish to explore sexual problems with your health care team.

Altered appearance, real or imagined, is one important barrier. Avoiding intimacy, thereby forestalling rejection, is a common response to feeling physically unattractive. The false belief that disabled people do not need or enjoy sex is widespread. It is true, however, that chronic illness affects self-image and self-confidence, and, like physical appearance, may lead to avoidance of intimacy. Partners, too, have problems, the most common of which is fear that intercourse may actually hurt their mate. This again may lead to a chain reaction of crossed signals.

It is important to know that intercourse is only a part of love. RA impacts on the whole family. Any loving mate suffers when you suffer, feels guilty for being well, and feels powerless when he or she can't help. Remaining or becoming close to one another is important to both partners. Imagine that you are young and dating. Get dressed, set a nice table, have good food, light candles, and play romantic music. You'll both feel better.

◆ CHAPTER ◆

15

Jeremiah J. Walsh: A Link Between RA's Past, Present, and Future

——◦◦(◦)◦◦——

This chapter is based on interviews and press releases conducted and written by Suzanne Loebl while science editor of the Arthritis Foundation. Even though the material dates from the 1970s, it is still pertinent because it emphasizes the courage of people suffering from RA. The story also illustrates the progression of arthritis knowledge during this past quarter of a century. And yet rheumatoid arthritis is still a miserable disease. All those suffering from it must have immense courage and determination, hoping, as Jerry Walsh did, that a permanent cure is just around the corner.

Jerry Walsh lived with RA for 34 years. Even though the disease kept him in bed for 8 years straight, he never let it dampen his spirits. In spite of his unremitting disease, it was hard to match Jerry's obvious joie de vivre.

Jerry was of Irish extraction, and though he was born in 1922 in Columbus, Ohio, he considered himself an Irishman. When Jerry was 14 years old, he won an athletic scholarship to Aquinas, a topnotch Catholic high school operated by the Dominican order in his hometown.

183

He did himself proud, and his achievements in sports, particularly baseball, won him local amateur and even professional fame. In 1940, Providence College offered him an athletic fellowship. At the time, he was also scouted by the Boston Red Sox, who considered him a potential major league baseball pitcher. A promising future lay ahead.

Fate would have it otherwise. During his last year in high school and first year in college, he began having pain and stiffness in his muscles and joints. His coaches, teammates, as well as Jerry himself, minimized these symptoms. For a long time, the disease he was suffering from had no name. It was variously considered as "growing pains" or a "muscle-bound" condition, which would disappear sooner or later.

Jerry claimed that he was advised to treat his condition by exercising. This he did, sometimes to excess and without benefit. Once when he was walking, or rather dragging himself around Columbus, the doctor who had taken care of him while he was on the Aquinas team drove past him and noted the trouble he was having. The doctor stopped and promptly had Jerry admitted to a hospital—the first of numerous other hospitalizations to follow.

At first, Jerry's condition was diagnosed as rheumatic fever. Later, as he recalled, "the doctor changed his mind and said that it was arthritis." He told Jerry's mother to "take me home and make me as comfortable as possible, for I would probably be in bed for the rest of my life, because there is nothing that anyone can do for arthritis." Various remedies were nevertheless tried. At one time, he was imprisoned in a full-length cast, which occasionally burst because his body and joints swelled up. The cast probably contributed to Jerry's physical deterioration. Jerry also developed psoriasis, which plagued him for the rest of his life.

Jerry was not resigned to staying in bed. Like most arthritics, he started to avail himself of every quack remedy that came his way: X-ray therapy, iodized water, electric devices, an oxydoner, 24 hours spent in a compost heap—you name it, Jerry did it. His disappointment and the rage he felt at being defrauded were the seeds from which eventually would grow his life's work. But that was far in the future.

In his search for help, he heard that "they knew something about arthritis at the Mayo Clinic in Rochester, Minnesota." Jerry was by then operating a greeting card business from his bed and started saving money. In 1944, he was on his way to Rochester. The trip was long and arduous. His stretcher was put aboard a train, and on the way he spent a day in the hospital of the railroad station in Chicago.

During the 1940s, the doctors at Mayo indeed "knew something about arthritis," but not enough. Jerry Walsh received aspirin, started a program of physical therapy, and was treated for his psoriasis. Jerry started to improve, but his hips were ankylosed (fused) and it would take years before he would learn how to stand.

At Mayo, Jerry started to form a close friendship with Dr. Howard Polley, who worked with Dr. Hench when the latter used corticosteroids to "cure" rheumatoid arthritis. Polley was also from Columbus. He had grown up across the street from Jerry's close friend, Jerry O'Shaughnessy, the son of the local undertaker. During his bedridden days, whenever Jerry Walsh had to go someplace, an O'Shaughnessy hearse would take him. Jerry O'Shaughnessy had delivered Jerry Walsh to the train that took him to Mayo, and the hearse again came to the station to pick him up when he returned.

Whenever he could, Jerry would go back to Mayo. All told, he must have spent years at the place. He grew to love the town, not only as he said "the mortar and bricks, but mostly the fact that the entire community was devoted to making people better." And the people in Rochester and at the Mayo Clinic grew to love Jerry. There was just something about Jerry Walsh that made people love and admire him: determination, courage, wit, and a great ability to understand and relate to others. There was only one thing that no one, least of all he, was allowed to do: feel sorry for Jerry Walsh. Everybody loved him wherever he went, and whenever he came back to Mayo, the message quickly traveled around the hall: "Jerry is back."

When he returned in 1951, cortisone had appeared on the medical horizon. Dr. Herman H. Young, another Ohio native, was Mayo's leading hip surgeon. Young agreed to operate on Jerry's hips if Jerry could come up with a 6-month supply of cortisone or ACTH (adrenocorticotrophic hormone). At the time, the drug was extracted from the adrenal glands of cattle and was a very rare commodity.

Jerry was fortunate. One of his numerous aunts worked for the Armor Company in Chicago, and within a few days, Jerry was assured of a continuous supply.

Dr. Young wanted to do only one of Jerry's hips and then have him recuperate at home. At the time, the operation consisted of separating the bones and inserting a metal cup into the acetabulum (the cup-shaped end of the pelvic bone). Jerry, with his ability to convince people to do anything, talked Dr. Young into doing the two hips during one hospital stay. Jerry had come to Mayo in January 1951 his usual way, via train and stretcher. He returned home on October 13, by air. When he stepped off the plane, Columbus cheered.

"My mother," Jerry recalled, "had seen me in bed for so many years that she suggested that if it hurt too much or was too difficult, I should not get up. But I had spent so much money trying to get up, and now that I had gotten up, I had to get out on my own and make it. But," he added, "it took me some time to emerge from horizontal hibernation and wear a business suit instead of pajamas."

In due time, he met Anne Crawford and got married. He wanted children, but proved infertile, probably as a consequence of X ray treatments. Anne and Jerry adopted Jimmy and Mary, two wonderful children to love and be loved by. Jerry Walsh also started to work for the Arthritis Foundation, first as a volunteer, then as a full-time staff member.

Jerry was ideally suited for the job. As one of his old friends said, "Jerry's philosophy was disarmingly simple. He was a special friend of every person suffering from arthritis. He knew their pain, their frustration, their humiliation, because they had been his all his adult life. Never was there a more articulate voice for the patient, never a more tireless worker, often exhausting staff and volunteers with his nonstop schedule when he toured America on behalf of the Arthritis Foundation. But Jerry was a happy crusader, full of wit and a bit of blarney, using his handicaps to tell the world what arthritis really is."

He was a gifted public speaker, and his special interest was attacking quackery. Wherever he went, he carried a "quack bag" containing useless devices that had been developed for sale to arthritis patients. The fact that he was so obviously handicapped was a door opener. As he liked to say, "A cripple never lies."

By posing as a potential customer, he started to help the government chase down some of the most egregious offenders. In 1963, Jerry Walsh testified in Washington before the Senate Subcommittee on Aging, which was investigating the Frauds and Quackery Affecting Older Citizens. The hearings were broadcast and televised, and Jerry Walsh became a national figure overnight. In the weeks that followed his testimony, he received 20,000 letters. To Jerry's great sorrow, most of these letters requested the addresses of the hucksters who sold the devices that he had just described as fraudulent.

In 1963, the President's Committee on Handicapped Americans nominated Jerry Walsh to be the Handicapped American of the Year. Before the honor was bestowed, President Kennedy was assassinated, and the award was presented the following March by President Lyndon B. Johnson.

Jerry really appreciated the honor not only for himself but also for the many kindred patients he represented. Jerry went to Washington with his entire family. Among the guests who attended the ceremony were members of Courage Incorporated, a self-help organization of physically challenged persons that Jerry had helped found during his bedridden days in Columbus.

It would be nice to say that Mayo "fixed Jerry up for good." But Jerry's rheumatoid arthritis continued with its ups and downs. He kept having serious flares, and at no time was he ever free of pain.

His hips reankylosed and he got around with a characteristic swing-through of the crutches. His left hand was almost totally deformed, the middle finger sticking into outer space. In typical Jerry Walsh fashion, he delighted in showing it to the barmen at the many hotels in which he stayed during his travels for the Arthritis Foundation, saying, "Look, I just caught my hand in your door." He claimed that this joke earned him an innumerable number of free drinks.

Jokes were a front, and at age 50 Jerry decided to have another go at his arthritis. In his travels for the Arthritis Foundation, he consulted several top-notch orthopedic surgeons and finally decided to try the Charnley-type hip replacement (see Chapter 16). The new implants were again to be put in at Mayo during the summer of 1975 by Dr. Mark Coventry, who had done more total hip replacement operations than any other U.S. surgeon. Jerry also had his hand fixed.

Dr. Coventry wanted to send Jerry home in between hip operations. Jerry, however, once more prevailed on having both hips and one hand done during a single hospitalization. The operations were a success. For the first time in more than 30 years, Jerry Walsh was entirely free of pain.

He went about the strenuous physical therapy routine in his customary way, and about 10 days after the second operation, Jerry recalled that he "was again walking like other people walk." That evening, he was so overwrought with emotion that he cried for 2 solid hours. Then he called Anne in New York to give her the good news.

Jerry returned to New York, but his luck had run out. About a month after his return, while he was alone at home, he tripped over a telephone cord and fell. In trying to catch himself, he grabbed at a chest of drawers, which fell on top of him. His leg, weakened by osteoporosis, was badly fractured. He was hospitalized at Columbia Presbyterian Hospital in New York.

The leg took 4 months to heal, and then there was a difference in the length of the legs. With further determination, Jerry was finally walking without a crutch.

But the pleasure would be only short-lived. On his last visit to Mayo, it was discovered that Jerry had leukemia. For 2 years, the malignancy was kept in check, but in the end the cancer overcame him.

As he would have wished, Jerry died with his boots on. On Monday afternoon, he delivered a luncheon speech for the Arthritis Foundation at Lenox Hill Hospital in New York City. He was ill. He had not eaten for days. Anne took him to St. Luke's Medical Center in New York. By Friday, he was sleeping all the time, and he died peacefully in his sleep on Tuesday night, November 11, 1975.

As he had requested, his funeral was in Columbus. A wake was held at the funeral home operated by Jerry Walsh's old friend, Jerry O'Shaughnessy, who had provided him with free transportation in the 1940s when he was bedridden. Seeing that there was actually an O'Shaughnessy Funeral Home almost seemed spooky to those who for years had listened to Jerry's stories.

In spite of the family's request to send donations to the Arthritis Foundation instead of flowers, the home was filled with roses. The funeral mass was held in St. Patrick's Cathedral, a Dominican church close to where old Aquinas had stood. The vicar of the church was a former umpire of Jerry's old baseball team. Father George Foucher, a grade-school friend of Jerry's, gave the eulogy.

To the many who had come to bid Jerry farewell, Father Foucher said, "Jerry would have told you: 'Sure, shed a tear for me, but go on living. Life is there to be enjoyed to the fullest despite any handicaps.'"

Around the time of his death in 1975, Jerry said, "I wish that I would know that my son, Jimmy, or anybody for that matter, will never have to suffer the way I did." Now, a quarter of a century later, his hopes are half true.

Treatment is much better than it was. Nobody today stays in bed for 8 years. Splints and physical therapy often prevent major deformities. Drug therapy has improved. Instead of a single DMARD (gold), which Jerry could not tolerate, there are a dozen. Surgery has come to the rescue for those whose joints need replacement. But RA and psoriasis are still with us. Let us wish that you are the last generation that must struggle with this severe disease. With luck and perseverance, new drugs will improve treatment. And perhaps a better understanding of genetic predisposition and of the immune system will soon yield a vaccine for those at risk of developing RA.

Extraordinary advances have occurred in our understanding and treatment of RA in recent years. Often, physicians can now identify patients they believe are likely to develop severe inflammation and treat them with more aggressive, yet safe, multidrug regimens. In addition, specific, narrowly focused immunological therapies have been developed and are now in widespread use. These medications target the major body chemicals that cause RA and joint damage. More than 60 percent of patients suffering from RA respond to these drugs with improved function and a decrease in permanent joint damage. The advent of sophisticated molecular, genetic, immunological, and other technological developments may enable scientists to identify those at risk of RA and rid them of the immune cells responsible for the onset of the disease. Perhaps then, as Jerry Walsh hoped, nobody ever will have to suffer the way he did.

16

Surgery and RA

This chapter reviews the development of total joint replacement, examines issues to consider before deciding on whether to have surgery, and discusses ways of locating a good surgeon/hospital combination. This chapter also presents information on how to prepare yourself and your home for orthopedic surgery, anesthesia, preadmission procedures, initial pain control after surgery, and respiratory exercises.

Jerry Walsh was among the first to receive new hips. Indeed, during the 1970s, the operating room became a new frontier for patients suffering from severe arthritis—and for many others whose joints had become non-functional for a variety of reasons. The total hip, the first major joint to be successfully replaced, was developed by Sir John Charnley in Brighton, England.

A look at the hip indicates that it is a rather simple joint. The ball-shaped end of the joint fits into in the *acetabulum*—the cup-like depression of the pelvis. It seemed rather simple to design a partial or total synthetic prosthesis. For years, some surgeons had attempted to repair hips by inserting a metal cup into the acetabulum. A total prosthesis would involve replacing the head of the femur with a ball and the acetabulum with a cup. There were several major challenges:

- Having the surfaces of the joint effortlessly slide over one another
- Affixing the parts of the joints to the wet, slippery surfaces of the body
- Once inserted, preventing the parts from loosening and/or wearing down when impacted by normal physical activity
- Avoiding infections of the replaced joint

Dr. Charnley resolved these problems one by one.

- Instead of using a metal-to-metal interface for the two parts of the joint, Charnley used synthetic polymer for one half, and a metal alloy for the other half. The resulting motion was smooth and effortless. Charnley made the cup part of the hip joint from Teflon, a polymer with excellent low-friction properties. Teflon, however, wore down quickly during normal usage, and after 300 failed hips, Charnley switched to the high-density polyethylene, which has been commonly used ever since. Today, both sides of a joint are made from a titanium alloy, but one half is lined with high-density polyethylene.
- Charnley resolved to cement the components of the synthetic joint onto, or into, healthy bone. Finding a material that would set rapidly in a moist environment was another hurdle. Methylmethacrylate cement was dentistry's suitable gift to joint replacement surgery.
- Attachment of the prosthesis to bone varies from joint to joint. In the case of the hip, long-lasting stability is derived by attaching the new femoral head to a long stem, which is then cemented into the hulled-out femur.
- Paying close attention to sterile conditions in the operating room minimized infections during total joint replacement. At HSS, the body of the patient is enclosed in a chamber filled with filtered air. The surgeons insert their hands through special openings.

Charnley's successful development of the total hip spurred the development of other total joints. Today, there are total joints for knees, elbows, shoulders, wrists, and even ankles. Some of these operations are detailed in Chapters 17, 18, and 19.

SURGICAL PROCEDURES USED
FOR PATIENTS SUFFERING FROM RA

In addition to total joint replacements, the following less radical procedures are also used.

Arthroscopy

An arthroscope, as its name implies, is used to look (*scope*) inside a joint (*arthro*). This small pencil-sized fiber-optic instrument is used for both diagnosis and minor surgery. Arthroscopes are used for small repairs (removal of debris or cartilage) as well as for removal of an inflamed synovium (synovectomy).

Synovectomy

The surgical removal of an inflamed synovium—especially of the knee— offers pain relief and improves function. The procedure, however, does not prevent cartilage loss. Regrowth of the synovial membrane often occurs within 3 to 5 years.

Osteotomy

Osteotomy is Greek for "cutting bone," and the procedure refers to realigning a joint, thereby restoring pain-free function.

Arthrodesis

This procedure involves the fusion of two bones, thereby eliminating pain and increasing stability. Today, the technique is mostly used to fuse ankles, wrists, vertebrae, and failed knee replacements.

COMPLICATIONS OF TOTAL JOINT REPLACEMENT

Total joint replacement surgery has become routine. The vast majority of the operations proceed without complications. Still, complications do occur. Major short-term complications include failed prostheses, infections, and development of embolisms (blood clots). Such complications often involve removal of the prosthesis, treatment of the infection, and reinsertion of the prosthesis. Prostheses also wear out. A hip prosthesis is expected to last about 15 to 20 years. Worn-out prostheses are replaced by new ones. The replacement of a prosthesis is called a *revision*. Given present-day technology, revisions are usually successful. In exceptional cases, they may require the fusion of a particular joint.

SHOULD YOU HAVE SURGERY?

Dr. Thomas Sculco, director of orthopedic surgery and the chief of Surgical Arthritis Services at HSS, considers surgery for patients suffering from RA "basically a last resort." When meeting a new patient, he carefully evaluates what the surgery will accomplish. For instance, will replacing a hip destroyed by RA protect the patient's other healthier hip? Will the surgery lessen unbearable pain? Will the operation restore the person's independence? Surgery should never be undertaken lightly. Here are factors that you must consider before undertaking any major surgical intervention.

Pain

Pain relief is one of the principal reasons for having surgery. As soon as Jerry Walsh woke up from the surgery, he realized that for the first time in 30 years his hip was no longer hurting. A level of pain that interferes with your sleep and your enjoyment of life is a valid reason for surgery.

What Will the Operation Accomplish?

Before answering, ask yourself: How much does your arthritic joint interfere with work and play? Would an operation make you more independent and self-reliant, enable you to work, shop, drive a car, or play cards? Are your joints unstable and do they present a hazard? An ankle fusion, for instance, may improve your overall stability and reduce the risk of falls.

Number of Joints Affected

Since RA affects more than one joint, discuss the order in which these joints should be repaired with your physician. Surgery involving the weight-bearing joints may require functional shoulders and elbows, to help navigate after the surgery.

Overall Health

The surgery will impact your other health problems. You may, for instance, suffer from heart disease. Will joint surgery stress your ailing heart, or will your repaired joints enable you to exercise and thereby improve your cardiovascular fitness?

Cost of Surgery

Surgery is expensive. Will your health insurance cover the cost? Will it cover other costs associated with surgery such as rehabilitation, equipment that you may need during rehabilitation, home care, transportation to and from the hospital, or possible loss of income?

Other Health Problems

Orthopedic procedures require vigorous rehabilitation. Do you feel that you will be strong enough to carry out the prescribed exercises?

Risk

Any type of surgery involves risk. This risk may be increased in the case of RA because:

◆ Extended corticosteroid therapy may have weakened the bone to which the prosthesis will be anchored. This may complicate the surgery and increase the risk of prosthetic loosening.

◆ Prolonged immunosuppressive therapy increases the risk of infection.

◆ Anesthesia may be more difficult because RA is a systemic disease sometimes associated with decreased pulmonary function.

◆ Rehabilitation of the new joint may be more difficult because of multiple joint involvement.

MAXIMIZING SUCCESS

Once you have decided that surgery is your best option, you should maximize your chances of success.

Getting a Second Opinion

Today, most health insurance companies require a second opinion before agreeing to pay for major surgery. Your physician will welcome a second opinion. Do not hesitate to ask him or her for a referral. Getting a second opinion will help you make this important decision.

Choosing Your Surgeon

Surgery has become highly specialized, and you will want to select a surgeon who is highly experienced in replacing or repairing your particular joint. Most often, but not always, the hospital and the surgeon go together. Physicians, including surgeons, are affiliated with particular hospitals. Sometimes, however, a surgeon may work at two different hospitals.

Choosing Your Hospital

For your joint replacement you should select a hospital that has a good rehabilitation department (physical therapy, occupational therapy) and is capable of handling emergencies (cardiac complications, infections) should they arise. Be aware that by selecting the most suitable surgeon/hospital combination, you may have to temporarily abandon your trusted physician (rheumatologist, primary care physician). As explained, physicians may only care for patients at hospitals with which they are affiliated. Your doctor may not necessarily have privileges at the orthopedic hospital of your choice.

While in the orthopedic hospital, you may be assigned to a doctor who is knowledgeable about the medical aspects related to orthopedic surgery. After discharge, you will return to your personal physician.

Talking to Another Patient

While deciding whether to have a particular operation, it is most helpful to talk to someone who had a similar procedure. Ask your doctor or surgeon for the telephone number of a suitable patient.

Getting a Start on Rehabilitation

It is best to undergo any type of surgery when you are in good shape. Ask your physician or physical therapist what type of exercises you can do before surgery to speed up your recovery.

Selecting an Appropriate Time for the Surgery

Hospital stays have been shortened to the minimum. Currently, the stay for an uncomplicated total hip is 4 to 5 days. In the mid-1980s, the stay for the same procedure was 2 weeks. Plan your surgery for a time when a friend or family member can help you recover at home.

Other considerations may dictate the timing of your surgery. Select a time that interferes least with your professional or other activities. Ask yourself whether it is best to have the surgery during the school year or in the summer. Do you want to recover in your garden when the weather is nice or in winter when you don't miss the outdoor fun?

GETTING READY

Once you have decided that you will have surgery, you must prepare for it. As in other aspects of your care, you remain the captain of your health team. In order to help patients fulfill that role, Suzanne Graziano, a nurse and patient educator at HSS, has organized classes for patients undergoing surgery there. During the class, patients learn what to expect before, during, and after surgery. Many of the suggestions provided in this and the following chapters are gleaned from this course.

HSS's hip and knee class is given several times a week. The classroom is equipped with a hospital bed. Each patient is given an imposing folder and an inspirometer (see below). Suzanne Graziano and her co-workers demonstrate how to get in and out of bed.

Medical Preparation

You should have a complete medical examination by your personal internist with special emphasis on the evaluation of your heart, circulatory and respiratory systems, and kidney function. Infections of any kind (e.g., skin, genitourinary tract) must be identified and treated. Visit your dentist to make sure that all existing or potential sources of oral infections are identified and treated.

A battery of general medical tests precedes any major surgical intervention. In addition, there may be tests for your specific procedure. Because same-day surgery is now usual, you will be evaluated a week or so prior to the actual surgery, most often in a special area of the hospital. During this evaluation, you may have an electrocardiogram (ECG), lab tests, X rays, pulmonary function evaluation, blood pressure measurements, and numerous other tests. You will sign forms and receive a copy of the "Patient's Bill of Rights." Among your other rights, this bill explains the procedure you must follow if you feel that your in-patient stay needs to be extended beyond the time recommended by the hospital.

Blood Transfusions

Anemia often occurs after total joint surgery, especially after hip and knee replacement. Some 20 years ago, patients routinely received blood from the blood bank that was collected from anyone willing to donate it. But with the arrival of AIDS and the prevalence of hepatitis, the risk of receiving contaminated blood increased for a while. Today, America's blood supply is much safer, but mishaps of the past have spurred the concept of autologous blood transfusions (donating your blood before, and in preparation for, the surgery).

Donating your own blood is a safe procedure because a healthy body manufactures new blood very quickly. Age is not a limiting factor. Provided they are in good health, elderly patients can donate their blood as successfully as young patients.

The following information about autologous blood transfusions will be useful:

♦ Find out from your surgeons how much blood will be required during the surgery (usually 1 to 2 pints for a total hip or knee).

♦ Discuss whether you should take iron supplements (300 mg three times per day is usual).

♦ Begin planning your autologous blood donation 4 to 6 weeks prior to surgery. It is usual to give 1 pint of blood during each donation. Except in emergencies, no blood is collected during the 72 hours prior to surgery.

♦ Eat breakfast if your blood donation is in the morning, or breakfast and lunch if your appointment is in the afternoon. Avoid eating fatty foods.

♦ Each blood donation takes about 20 minutes.

LEGAL MATTERS, RED TAPE, AND PAPERWORK

Insurance

Insurance companies are very particular about reimbursement procedures. Read your contract with your insurance company very carefully to see what kind of preauthorization is needed in each case. Obtain all required preauthorizations. Read your contract to determine whether the following items are covered: physical therapy, private-duty nursing, medications, assistive devices (canes, crutches, toilet seat, other), stays at rehabilitation centers, and home health care.

The Social Service Department or patient care coordinator of the hospital at which you have your surgery may help you understand your contract and/or assist you in obtaining additional coverage.

Health Care Proxy and Advanced Directives

Unless you have done so previously, appoint your partner, friend, or relative to make appropriate medical decisions should you be unable to do so.

Surgical Informed Consent Form

This form is meant to inform you about the reasons for and potential side effects related to the proposed surgery. Once you have read it and received answers to your questions, you will have to sign a form authorizing the surgery and indicating that you understand the risks. You may file this form ahead of time or bring it with you on the day of the surgery.

Bills

Pay all your outstanding or predictable bills before you enter the hospital. Arrange to pay your rent, credit card, and telephone bills while in the hospital. Do banking in advance if possible.

PREPARING YOUR HOME

You will be handicapped and tired when you return home from the hospital. The recommended modification of your quarters will depend on the specific type of surgery you underwent. Here are some general suggestions on how to speed up your recovery:

◆   Arrange to have someone stay with you during the initial weeks after surgery.

◆   Make your home slip-proof. Remove throw rugs, clutter, and small objects so that you can move about freely. When you get home, avoid stumbling over your pet.

- Place necessary items within easy reach. Have a cordless phone to carry with you.

- Make sure that you can easily maneuver in your bathroom. Postpone showering until sutures and staples have been removed. If you had hip surgery, use a raised toilet seat and a stall shower.

- Prepare meals ahead of time and store in the freezer. Stock up on staples and frozen dinners. Have phone numbers of favorite home delivery foods handy. Arrange for Meals on Wheels to deliver food if necessary. Ask your friends to visit and bring dinner.

- Arrange for suitable furniture. Hip patients should buy, borrow, or rent a high chair with arms. Alternatively, put two pillows on a firm ordinary chair.

- The enforced rest after joint replacement surgery is a rare opportunity to do projects you are usually too busy for—for example, pasting in photographs, writing to friends, or listening to music. Also, stock up on books, magazines, handicrafts, videotapes, and jigsaw puzzles.

GOING TO THE HOSPITAL

In the new same-day surgery routine (see below) the patient assumes responsibility for some important preoperative procedures.

Cleaning Out Your Gut

Some surgeons or hospitals require you to empty your gastrointestinal (GI) tract before anesthesia is administered and surgery is performed; others do not.

- On the day prior to surgery, maintain a liquid diet consisting of clear soups, Jell-O, custard, yogurt, ice cream, and cold cereals.

- In the evening, a couple of hours after dinner, give yourself an enema with a ready-to-use kit from your local drugstore.

- In order to eliminate the risk of aspirating food particles during anesthesia, it is crucial that your digestive system be completely empty. Unless otherwise instructed by your physician, do not eat, drink, or take any medications after midnight the night before surgery. Patients with diabetes or other metabolic disorders must discuss these instructions with their physician.

◆ Do not take aspirin or NSAIDs for at least 1 week prior to surgery to avoid problems with bleeding.

Packing for the Hospital

Don't take much. The hospital will provide sleepwear. Leave valuables, personal treasures, jewelry, and credit cards at home. Bring the following items:

◆ Paperwork, including surgical consent form, health care proxy, X-ray and lab reports (if requested).

◆ Telephone numbers of people you may want to call.

◆ Cane or crutches, if applicable. Physical therapists will adjust or re-adjust their height.

◆ Flat, supportive athletic or walking shoes with nonskid soles. Bring orthotics, if you use them.

◆ Short nightgown or loose pajamas (optional).

◆ Short lightweight bathrobe (short clothing prevents tripping while walking).

◆ Personal toiletries, makeup, electric razor.

◆ Eyeglasses (hospital staff recommends leaving contact lenses at home because they get lost easily).

◆ Dentures.

◆ Bring a list of all the medications you take regularly including those you have not been taking in anticipation of surgery. Bring medications that you think the hospital may not have on hand, especially eyedrops or inhalers. However, do not take any medication on your own. Make sure that hospital personnel (physicians, nurses) are aware of your needs. Getting too much or not enough medication can have grave consequences. When you discuss these medications with the hospital staff, ascertain that they are aware of any drug allergies you may have.

◆ Small amount of cash ($20) for newspapers and other small items.

◆ A book, magazine, inexpensive battery-operated radio, relaxation tapes. If possible, ask your visitors to bring these items after your surgery.

◆ Sweatsuit or loose-fitting clothes to wear when going home.

◆ A sleep mask and ear plugs.

IF YOU HAVE SAME-DAY SURGERY

Because of the escalating cost of surgery, you may arrive on the day on which you will have your surgery. You will arrive at the hospital about 3 hours prior to the surgery. You will enter a special same-day surgery suite, don hospital garb, undergo a physical and possibly a few tests. The in-depth surgical evaluation was done while you were an outpatient. You will then be transferred to the operating room.

ANESTHESIA

Surgery as we know it today owes part of its growth to the discovery of anesthesia. Since the early days, anesthesia has become a major branch of medicine, and the anesthesiologist—a highly trained physician—is a crucial member of the surgical team. He or she will meet you during your preoperative assessment or in the same-day surgery admissions unit. The anesthesiologist will completely review your medical history and will ask specific questions about drug allergies and your prior surgical and anesthetic history. He or she will discuss the options regarding the type of anesthesia that best fits your needs.

Many people are afraid of general anesthesia, fearing that they may never wake up. The best antidote to fear is knowledge, so here are a few facts, many of them derived from the excellent booklet, "Removing the Mystery from Regional Anesthesia," which is part of the Patient Education Series developed by HSS.

Anesthetic drugs are narcotics that eliminate pain and can induce sleep. These drugs vary in length of action. Some, like those administered during tooth extraction, are very short-acting. Others last longer. During a long surgical procedure, the anesthesiologist monitors the amount of drug you need at any one time. The anesthesiologist evaluates the depth of the anesthesia, your respiration, heart rate, blood pressure, and other vital functions, intervening when necessary.

Before you enter the operating room, you will be sedated and you will drift into twilight sleep.

Anesthesia can be either general or regional. General anesthesia, which numbs the entire body, is administered through a breathing tube attached to a respirator that also delivers oxygen from a tube inserted through the trachea (windpipe). The advantage of general anesthesia is that it eliminates all awareness of the surroundings. The disadvantage is that pain and other sensations return once the anesthesia wears off. In addition, sore throats, nausea, vomiting, and "hangovers" commonly occur after general anesthesia.

Regional anesthesia is preferred for orthopedic surgery. The recovery from this type of anesthesia is quicker and the transition to selective pain control is smoother. Regional anesthesia usually eliminates use of a breathing tube. It totally eliminates pain in a given region of your body.

During regional anesthesia, even though you are technically awake, you will not remember much, though you are aware of your surroundings and hear the ongoing conversation. You may even be able to ask or answer questions. You will not see the operation because your head is separated from the surgical site by sterile drapes and other paraphernalia. If this bothers you, ask your anesthesiologist to put you to sleep with a mild sedative. Then you will wake up in the recovery room.

Regional anesthesia blocks out selected nerve paths, permitting surgeons to operate on all parts of your body: hands, feet, knees, and hips.

Two regional techniques are used for surgery below the abdomen (hips and knees): spinal anesthesia and epidural anesthesia, each having minor advantages and disadvantages. During spinal anesthesia, the anesthetic is injected directly into the lumbar spinal canal with a very fine needle, which is then withdrawn postoperatively. Spinal anesthesia is used for lower limb surgery. It has few side effects (only 1 percent of patients suffer from spinal headaches). The anesthesia, however, lasts only 2 hours, and if surgery is prolonged, additional doses of anesthetics are required.

During epidural anesthesia, the anesthetic is injected outside the dura mater (the tough membrane that surrounds the spinal fluid). The anesthetic is delivered to the appropriate spot through a very thin tube, which remains in place during surgery. This permits the anesthesiologist to administer additional anesthetic if the surgery lasts more than 2 to 2 1/2 hours. The procedure is associated with a slightly higher incidence of back soreness and backaches. The incidence of spinal headaches is 0.5 percent. A still newer technique combines spinal and epidural anesthesia by using the thin needles used during spinal anesthesia inside a correctly placed epidural needle, which stays in place during surgery.

Anesthesia for surgery involving the upper limbs (shoulders, arms, hands) requires the injection(s) of anesthetic where it will block sensation transmitted to specific groups of nerves. Common techniques and sites include a brachial plexus block, an interscalene block, and an axillary block. The anesthetic effect lasts 4 to 5 hours. An ankle block, whose effect lasts from 3 to 24 hours, is used for foot surgery. The surgical procedures are covered in Chapters 17, 18, and 19.

RECOVERY

After the surgical procedure, you will be moved to the postanesthesia care unit (PACU), formerly known as the recovery room. You may be provided with oxygen, which speeds up the healing process, and intravenous lines. Your cardiac and respiratory function will be carefully monitored. The blood you donated may be returned to you, unless this was done in the operating room. Most patients stay in the recovery for 3 to 5 hours.

Once you are fully awake, you will notice the bulky dressing that surrounds your newly operated joint, and the tubes that may drain fluid from your wound or urine from your bladder. Oxygen may be delivered through a thin plastic tube entering your nose. Another plastic tubing, entering the vein on your arm, will deliver fluids containing glucose, lactated Ringer's solution or saline, as well as antibiotics. You will try to lie comfortably, but chances are that the positions you can assume are dictated by the surgery. Hip patients are tethered to their bed, their leg in a sling. You may feel helpless and vulnerable, but the nurses will attempt to make you as comfortable as possible.

Surgery is very stressful. You will be exhausted. The pain emanating from your arthritic joint may have diminished, but your surgical wound, your back, your head, and various muscle groups may hurt.

Except for diagnostic purposes or as a warning sign, pain fulfills no useful purpose. Hospital staff will help you reduce your postoperative pain. Pain is very personal and difficult to measure. There is no need for you to brave pain. Mild pain is easier to control than severe pain. Do not wait until your pain is unbearable before telling the nurse that you need help. During the first day or two after surgery, the pain-control medication will be injected; thereafter, it will be administered orally.

Some hospitals, including HSS, use a special apparatus that allows patients to control their own pain. Patient-controlled anesthesia (PCA) enables you to inject yourself with small doses of pain medication whenever you hurt (Fig. 16-1). The device consists of a little battery-operated pump and tubing that delivers medication (morphine, Marcaine, other) directly to your spinal cord (epidural) or intravenously. The device is safe—it has been programmed not to deliver an overdose. Also, there is no danger of developing an addiction. The pain-relieving ability of ice packs is not to be underestimated. It is best to apply these to the surgical area for 20 minutes every 4 hours or four to five times/day. Continue to apply ice after you return home. See Chapter 14 for additional methods of pain relief.

FIGURE 16-1. The Patient-Controlled Anesthesia Device Used at the Hospital for Special Surgery. *From* Your Pathway to Recovery, *by Suzanne Graziano, Department of Nursing Administration, HSS.*

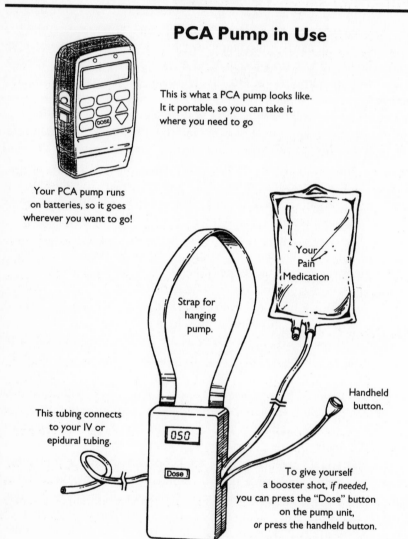

PCA Pump in Use

This is what a PCA pump looks like. It it portable, so you can take it where you need to go

Your PCA pump runs on batteries, so it goes wherever you want to go!

Your Pain Medication

Strap for hanging pump.

Handheld button.

This tubing connects to your IV or epidural tubing.

050

Dose

To give yourself a booster shot, *if needed*, you can press the "Dose" button on the pump unit, *or press the handheld button.*

Your Hospital Stay

Medical and Surgical Assessments

On a daily basis, your surgeon and internist will visit you to make sure that things are proceeding normally. They will focus on your wound, your temperature and vital signs, your heart, lung, bowel, and urinary function. Daily blood tests are common after joint replacement to monitor your health.

Private-Duty Nursing

Hospitals are busy places with a busy staff. During the initial days after surgery, you will feel quite helpless and uncomfortable, and it is nice to have someone who can quickly rearrange your pillow, bring you water, and even turn your radio on and off. If you can afford it, hire a nurse during the initial day(s) or night(s) after surgery. Since you are not really very sick, a practical nurse or a nursing aide, rather than a registered nurse, will do. When asked, the nursing office of the hospital will arrange for private-duty nursing.

Breathing Exercises

After surgery it is crucial that you exercise your lungs by breathing deeply. This not only improves blood oxygenation but also avoids the collapse of small areas of the lung, thereby preventing pneumonia. Normally, you automatically breathe deeply once or twice an hour. Anesthesia and pain upset this breathing pattern, and you must make a positive effort to exercise your lungs.

The plastic inspiromenter provided by the hospital consists of several chambers, each of which contains a small plastic ball (Fig. 16-2). Tubing connects the device to a mouthpiece. When not in use, the balls rest on the bottom of the chamber. When you extract the air by inhaling (inspirating), the balls rise to the top.

During the lung exercises, place the mouthpiece in your mouth. Exhale normally. Hold your breath to a count of five. Inhale slowly and deeply. The balls in the chamber rise to the top. Rest. Repeat, alternating between inhalations that raise one ball and those that raise two or three balls. Make a habit of using your inspirometer 10 times an hour during the first few days after surgery.

FIGURE 16-2. An Inspirometer. When used regularly, 10 times an hour while awake during the first days after surgery, an inspirometer promotes deep breathing. *From* Your Pathway to Recovery, *by Suzanne Graziano, Department of Nursing Administration, HSS.*

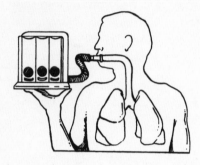

With the unit in an upright position, exhale normally; then place your lips tightly around the mouthpiece.

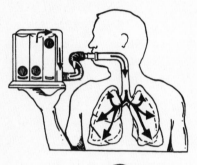

To achieve a slow Sustained Maximal Inspiration (SMI)...inhale at a rate sufficient to raise only the ball in the first chamber, while the ball in the second chamber remains at rest.

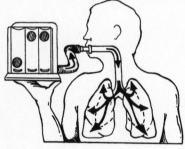

For a higher flow rate...

Inhale at a rate sufficient to raise the first and second balls, while the ball in the third chamber remains at rest.

Exhale...

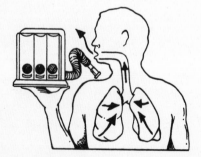

After performing exercise, remove the mouthpiece from your lips and exhale normally.

Then relax...

Following each prolonged deep breath, take a moment to rest and breathe normally.

A few days after surgery, you can make yourself cough to clear and exercise your lungs. Breathe in deeply through your nose, hold your breath to a count of five, and breathe out slowly through your mouth. On the fifth deep breath, cough from your abdomen as you breathe out. Repeat two or three times per hour, especially when not using your inspirometer.

Exercise

Physical therapy is an essential part of your postoperative recovery. Surgeons are very particular about which exercises should be done after surgery and when they should be done. The physical therapist will follow these instructions.

The types of exercise you will do are dictated by what joint was operated on. Patients with hip replacements are cautioned to never elevate their knee above the level of the hip (as you would when sitting in a deep armchair). Newly operated-on knees are bent within a day after the operation in a continuously passive motion machine. Suffice it to say that you will start exercising gently almost immediately after surgery and that it will seem very difficult. The muscles on your operated-on limb will seem weak. You'll worry about whether your new knee, or hip, can support you. You'll be very tired and you'll balk at being asked to pump your ankles, or tighten your quads and your butt, while trying to relax in bed.

The physical therapist will help you sit at the edge of your bed and dangle your feet. Then you will learn to stand, amble to your chair, sit, and eventually stand up again. Then you will take a few tentative steps. Within days, you'll walk down the hall. Never stand up directly before you have sat for a minute or so, dangling your feet. This gives your body a chance to adjust and prevents a sudden drop in blood pressure (orthostatic hypotension). Before discharge, you will go to the gym where you'll practice walking up and down stairs and getting in and out of a car.

Bladder and Bowel

A Foley catheter that drains the bladder is used for hip and knee surgery. It is usually removed after 24 to 48 hours. Initially, until getting out of bed is no longer a major undertaking, you'll use a bedpan.

Your bowels "go to sleep" when you undergo surgery and anesthesia. Thus, it may take some time—usually 3 to 4 days—until you have a bowel movement. The doctor or nurse will listen daily to your bowel sounds with a stethoscope and ask you if you have "passed gas," to determine whether you're producing intestinal gas, which is a sign of return of bowel function.

Food after Surgery

Chances are that you will not be hungry, which is just as well. Because of the bowel changes, on the day of the surgery you will only be allowed to suck on ice chips. The next day, you will receive what Suzanne Graziano describes as "the gourmet liquid tray" consisting of Jell-O, clear broth, and tea. On day 3, when the food service delivers real food, you will be almost ready to go home.

Blood Thinners (Anticoagulants)

Some patients undergoing joint replacement surgery develop clots in the veins of their thighs or calves. If these are found postoperatively, anticoagulant therapy may be prescribed in the hospital and after discharge. Coumadin is a commonly prescribed anticoagulant, and a usual course lasts 6 to 8 weeks. The medication requires close monitoring, which will be coordinated by your physician. For most patients, precautionary anticoagulant therapy simply consists of taking aspirin.

Occupational Therapy

After you have recovered somewhat and can navigate on your own, you may visit the occupational therapy department, where you will be taught how to protect your freshly operated joints (see also Chapters 17 and 18 for details). The occupational therapist will provide you with aids to daily living (ADLs) including long-handled shoehorns and tongs to pick objects off the floor, raised toilet seats, and so on. They will remind you of what you can and cannot do. The physical therapy or nursing staff often provides these instructions.

Case Management or Social Service Departments

A friend or relative using a private car or taxi can pick up most patients. (After total hip replacement, consult Table 18–1.) The hospital can also arrange for a private ambulette with attendants who assist patients up cumbersome stairs.

Experienced professionals will help you navigate through a sea of red tape as you deal with health insurance matters.

Because hospital stays are short, you will need a support structure after discharge. It is highly desirable that a family member or close friend be available to help you with routine chores during at least the first week following major surgery. If this cannot be arranged, discuss the situation with your physician, case manager, or social service department. Under your health insurance you may qualify for personal care assistance. If skilled care is not medically indicated, the case manager can usually provide the name(s) of qualified home health agencies.

If your particular medical circumstances warrant it, your physician may recommend that you be discharged to a rehabilitation hospital. If your physician anticipates such a need, it is best to explore this possibility before the actual surgery. Rehabilitation centers provide personal care as well as intensive physical therapy. If indicated, such arrangements can also be made after surgery.

It is crucial that you continue the physical rehabilitation of your new joint once you get home. Most often, patients can do exercises on their own after discharge provided that they follow the instructions provided by their medical team. Many medical insurances (Medicare, others) pay for home visits by physical therapists. Again, proper authorization (prescription from physician or surgeon, preauthorization from insurance provider) is required.

Patients may also require outpatient physical therapy. It can be provided by the hospital at which the surgery took place or by an independent physical therapy practice. To obtain reimbursement, you need a prescription from your surgeon and sometimes clearance from your insurance provider. You also will have to arrange for suitable transportation.

Discharge

Before leaving the hospital make sure that you:

- Have written instructions telling you what to do and what not to do.
- Have detailed prescriptions for pain and other medications.
- Have clear instructions about the rehabilitation exercises you should do, including how often and when. Most often, exercises should be done twice a day.

- ◆ Have phone numbers of your physician(s) should an emergency arise.

- ◆ Have the medications you brought to the hospital.

- ◆ Be certain you know how, where, and when to get blood tests that monitor your blood coagulation if you are taking Coumadin, and, if necessary, which doctor will adjust the dosage.

You will also be required to sign all kinds of discharge papers before leaving.

Once you are home, you will continue to feel tired. Go to bed as soon as you can. Continue to take your pain medication. Apply cold compresses and remember that *it is extremely important for you to do your rehabilitation exercises as instructed.* Soon you'll feel better. Read books, knit, do jigsaw puzzles and catch up on the other things you planned to do during your recovery.

17

Surgery of the Knee

═══◉═══

*This chapter reviews rheumatoid arthritis of the knee and follows a patient
during total knee replacement (TKR) surgery.*

RHEUMATOID ARTHRITIS OF THE KNEE

On the way to the grocery store, Vanessa B. stopped short. She realized
that she was actually smiling. She could not recall having smiled while
walking anywhere for years. Then she remembered her 4-month-old
knee. Perhaps she also thought of all the people who had made the miracle possible: scientists, physicians, surgeons, nurses, physical therapists,
her parents, friends, and colleagues, and, most of all, herself. Without
determination she would not have graduated from Mount Holyoke with
high honors. Now she is teaching second grade at one of Manhattan's
top private schools, where her students love her. Even on the phone, her
voice is happy.

Vanessa, now 26, belongs to the 10 percent of juvenile rheumatoid
arthritis (JRA) patients who fail to outgrow their disease. She developed
JRA when she was 2½ years old. Even then her knees were the principal focus of the disease. It was a constant struggle: the pain, the flares,
the tons of aspirin, and the traction. When asked how it felt to be chron-
ically ill as a child, she admits that her spirits were not always up. "High

school was bad." she said. "I had many flares and a lot of pain. It was difficult to talk about my disease to the other kids, because one could not really 'see' the arthritis. In college I did flare badly during the junior year, but by then I realized that it was my fault. I failed to listen to my body. For me that makes the difference between being ill or well." For Vanessa, paying attention to her body means not overdoing activities and getting 8 to 8½ hours of sleep at night.

After college, Vanessa returned to Manhattan. She took a year off and then started teaching school. Drs. Susan Goodman and Steven Magid of HSS's Department of Rheumatology kept her arthritis in check. "For years, I took Plaquenil," she says, "but I don't know whether it helped." Since it was approved, Vanessa takes Celebrex, the COX-2 inhibitor. She says, "It is good stuff." Walking, however, became increasingly painful and difficult. "I kept calculating: Can I walk these three blocks without resting or not? I had extreme trouble getting up out of a chair, and I even hesitated to go from one room to the next.

"I don't know whether I didn't hear my doctor saying that I was 'losing cartilage,' or whether she did not say clearly enough that I was in real trouble. But in January 1999, when Dr. Goodman told me that I needed a new knee, I went into shock. I did a lot of soul searching as to whether to have the operation or not," Vanessa continued. "I finally realized that I could not possibly go through another painful, handicapped year like the last one. I decided to have the operation. I was given the name of several surgeons and opted for Dr. Nestor because my insurance company approved him without a hassle. I was operated on in July."

Whereas many surgeons specialize in one or two joints. Dr. Nestor is unusual in that he operates on many different joints. "Since rheumatoid arthritis has an impact on many joints," Dr. Nestor says, "I focus on hips, knees, shoulders, and elbows."

THE OPERATING ROOM

It is 3:30 P.M. and Dr. Nestor is about to do a total knee replacement (TKR). The patient, a middle-aged man who we shall call Bob R., arrives in Operating Room (OR) #11 at HSS on a stretcher. He is fully awake and has chosen to remain awake during the entire procedure. He is transferred to the operating table and asked to sit up and bend forward. Dr. K., the anesthesiologist, repeatedly scrubs Bob R.'s back with Betadine, a brown iodine-containing antiseptic solution. Carefully, Dr. K. searches for the space between the vertebrae and injects a predetermined amount of anesthetic for regional anesthesia that will block pain in the leg. The actual operating time is estimated at 90 minutes. Dr. K. has allowed for ample leeway. There will be no sensation in the lower part of the body for approximately 2½ hours.

Under the supervision of the OR nurse, the OR is being set up for surgery. Extreme caution is taken to avoid sources of infection. Sliding Plexiglas panels are put in place, and this space is filled with filtered air. Anyone within this enclosure must wear a sterilized gown over familiar blue scrubs, a sort of space helmet over the head, and latex gloves.

In addition to Dr. K., five people will assist Dr. Nestor today: two surgical residents, two surgical technicians, and a registered nurse. The nurse is stationed outside the enclosure and is responsible for the team maintaining sterility throughout the procedure. One of the surgical assistants works closely with the medical team; the other hands dozens of instruments and supplies to the surgical team as needed. Together the team works as if it were a well-rehearsed orchestra. The registered nurse, referred to as the circulating nurse, supervises the preparation of the operating room, keeps accurate records, and retrieves supplies as needed.

As soon as Bob is anesthetized, the surgical team "preps" him. A sterile plastic sheet is fastened in such a manner that the patient's upper body is separated from the lower body. Intravenous lines are inserted into his arm to permit the delivery of fluid, blood, and antibiotics. The latter are administered routinely during total joint replacement to prevent infection. Bob is connected to monitoring devices and is constantly watched over by the anesthetist who is sitting next to his head. Bob's blood and pulmonary pressures, as well as his heart and pulse rate, are displayed on a screen. Bob also receives additional oxygen to help oxygenate his blood.

Bob's entire body, including the healthy leg, is wrapped in various sterile sheets. The leg that will be operated on is scrubbed with Betadine solution. A plastic sheet, lined with specially treated antiseptic, is pasted on the leg. It will remain in place throughout the entire operation.

Whenever possible, surgeons like to operate in a "bloodless field." Bob's lower leg and knee are temporarily wrapped into a big Ace bandage. The blood from the leg is compressed into the general circulation. Then a big tourniquet is strapped to the upper portion of the thigh to decrease blood flow into the leg during the operation. Nothing shows except for the knee and part of the lower leg. Dr. Nestor carefully examines the X rays of Bob's knee that are prominently displayed on a light box. He is ready to begin the operation.

ANATOMY OF THE KNEE

The Bony Structure

Unlike the hip, the human knee is not embedded in lots of muscle tissue. The knee connects the two longest bones of the body: the *femur,* or thighbone, and the *tibia,* or shinbone. A thinner bone, the *fibula,* runs along the tibia but is not part of the knee joint. The knee also includes a small, round bone, the *patella* or kneecap, which fits neatly into a grove (the *trochlea*) at the end of the femur. As shown in Figure 17–1, the ends of the femur and the tibia are intricately shaped. The end of the femur consists of two rounded knuckles, the *femoral condyles.* The tibia ends in a plateau, the *tibial plateau,* which is separated in the middle by the *tibial eminence.* The surfaces of the femur and the tibia are not matched perfectly. The *meniscus,* a rubbery shock-absorbing tissue, fits snugly between the two bones and improves contact.

The Soft Tissues

For mobility and stability, the knee relies on an intricate network of soft tissues.

The Ligaments

The ligaments keep the components of the knee in place. Five ligaments are particularly important: two *collateral ligaments,* which run on the outside and the inside of the knee, two *cruciate ligaments,* which cross inside the knee, and the *patellar ligament* (sometimes called the *patellar tendon*), which connects the patella to the tibia. Preserving these numerous tendons, which in concert are so important to the function of the knee, was one of the principal problems doctors encountered in developing a successful total knee prosthesis.

The Muscles

The principal muscles servicing the knee are the four *quadriceps,* the three *hamstrings,* and the *gastrocnemius.* The quadriceps run down the front of the thigh into the knee joint. The muscles straighten and bend the knee and maintain it in a locked position when bending over. The hamstrings run down the back and sides of the knee, and the gastrocnemius runs along the back of the knee. Together with the ligaments,

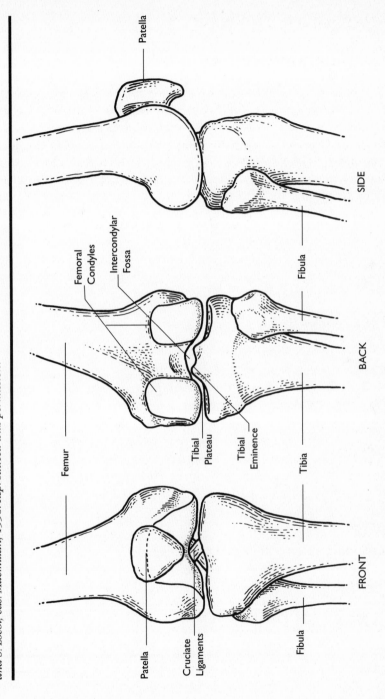

FIGURE 17-1. The Anatomy of the Knee. *From* The Columbia Presbyterian Osteoarthritis Handbook, *R. P. Grelsamer and S. Loebl, eds. Macmillan, 1996. Reproduced with permission.*

the rehabilitation of these muscles after surgery is the key to a good outcome.

The Meniscus

The rubbery menisci (actually there are two, though they are usually referred to as one unit), which take on the shape of the tibia and femur, are quite vulnerable and easily injured during sporting accidents. Today, tears in the meniscus are usually repaired by arthroscopy. During this procedure the surgeon smoothes and straightens the surface of the meniscus.

The Cartilage

As in all joints, the glossy, glass-like hyaline cartilage that covers the ends of the knee bones is essential for smooth movement. Rheumatoid arthritis singles out cartilage, causing it to become buckled, pitted, and eroded. It was the loss of cartilage and structural changes in the joint that finally sent Vanessa to the surgeon for a new knee.

The Joint Capsule

The knee is enclosed in a joint capsule lined by synovium. Inflammation of the synovium is an early finding in RA. This inflammation is accompanied by the secretion of fluid, swelling, pain, and discomfort. Excessive fluid is sometimes drained by a needle and a steroid-containing solution is injected into the knee to treat discomfort.

In the early stages of the disease after the synovium is inflamed but before the cartilage has been destroyed, a synovectomy (removal of the joint lining) is sometimes performed. This can provide pain relief and reduce swelling for 3 to 5 years.

Bursae

Numerous small fluid-filled sacs cushion ligaments and tendons throughout the knee. These bursae may become inflamed, causing bursitis.

FUNCTIONS OF THE KNEE

The knee is highly mobile. It can flex from 0° to 140°. It is not a simple hinge joint because it allows the tibia to swivel. When fully extended, the knee locks upon itself and becomes rigid.

The stability of the knee derives entirely from the ligaments and muscles that surround it. Any weakening of this supporting structure decreases stability.

The knee bears the entire weight of the body, which is effectively increased several-fold during walking and other daily activity. The elastic tissues of the knee (meniscus, cartilage) absorb some of this impact, as do the muscles that tighten when anticipating a step.

Ideally, the weight of the body follows a plumb line from the center of the hip to the center of the knee to the center of the ankle. Many people, however, are slightly bow-legged or knock-kneed, and, similar to an unbalanced automobile tire, portions of the knee, especially the condyles, wear unevenly. Wear and disease do not necessarily affect all parts of the knee evenly. As RA progresses, the malalignment amplifies until it reaches a critical point, when the knee becomes clearly nonfunctional. Like Vanessa, many other patients will tell you that they reached the decision to have their knee replaced rather suddenly.

THE DEVELOPMENT
OF THE TOTAL KNEE PROSTHESIS

Attempts at developing a total knee implant date from the 1940s. Designers faced two major difficulties: mimicking the complex mechanism of the knee and preserving the intricate soft tissue structure.

During the 1970s and 1980s, there was a plethora of artificial designs for knees—a sure sign that none of the designs were perfect. Finally, surgeons settled on the following overall design, which is now used universally. This total knee was developed at HSS and is known as the Insall-Burstein Condylar Design. As seen in Figure 17–2, the main portion of the prosthesis consists of:

◆   A one-piece femoral component in which two runners, connected by a short bar, fit over the end of the femur as if it were a huge dental cap. Each runner has a short stem on its underside that is cemented into the resected (cut-down) condyle. The prosthesis is called *bicondylar* because both condyles are rebuilt with one prosthesis.

◆   The tibial component, which consists of a high-density polyethylene plateau whose shallow tracks articulate (move together) smoothly with the runners of the femoral portion of the knee. A metal plateau,

FIGURE 17-2. A Total Knee Prosthesis. *From Wright Medical Technology, Inc.*

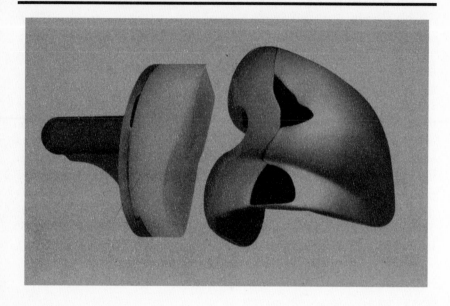

whose short stem will be cemented into the tibia, supports the plastic interface.

♦ The polyethylene "button" that replaces the patella (not shown).

When implanted, an artificial knee bends less than the person's own knee. The degree to which a replaced knee joint bends depends mainly on the strength and elasticity of the soft tissues surrounding the joint.

BACK TO THE OPERATING ROOM

After Bob R. is prepped, Dr. Nestor incises the skin. Taking care to push the ligaments aside, he separates the two halves of the joint. He first turns his attention to the tibia. It is shaved down, but not too much. He drills holes in the newly flat surface.

When he is satisfied with the surface of the tibia, he exposes the two condyles that form the lower end of the femur. Since the field is bloodless, it is easy to see that these knobs are a larger version of the familiar second joint of a chicken. Once nature has developed a good design, it uses it repeatedly. Carefully, Dr. Nestor cuts away the rounded condyles. All this takes a while.

The surgeons work intensely. During the procedure, you can hear the buzzing of an electric saw, the high-pitched humming of an electric scalpel, the banging of a hammer, and the tapping of a chisel. The team resembles a group of master carpenters.

Instruments are passed back and forth between the doctors and the surgical technician who is hovering over the instrument cases. Most of the time she knows what will be needed next before anyone asks for it. When something special is required, the circulating nurse obtains it from inventory outside the OR. When she returns with the item, she removes the outer nonsterile wrap and drops the now sterile object into the sterile enclosure without touching it.

The time has come to try the new prosthesis. Dr. Nestor asks for a test prosthesis. The two parts are inserted. The knee is bent, straightened, and twisted. Everybody is satisfied, and now it is time to insert the artificial joint.

The circulating nurse is asked to obtain three components from inventory: the tibial and femoral components and the patella. The code of each item is double-checked. The surgical team calls for two units of cement. This rapidly setting glue has to be mixed on the spot. The surgical technician hands it to her colleague, who stirs it a few minutes until it has a smooth consistency. Then the cement is applied to the prepared end of the femur; the new femoral component is inserted and finally hammered into place. It takes a few minutes for the cement to set. The tibial plateau is inserted in the same manner. Then it is the turn of the patella. The joint cavity is carefully cleaned. "We are closing," somebody calls out. It is 5:30 P.M. The preparation, induction of anesthesia, and operation has lasted 2 hours.

The various layers of tissue are sutured back together, ending with the skin. The surgical team continues to function as if it were a well-oiled machine. Curved needles are passed back and forth with forceps. The surgical technician threads the needles and the surgical team does the suturing, tying, and cutting of the thread after each stitch. It takes 10 minutes to close the long wound. A very thin plastic tubing is inserted into the surgical site. The purpose of this *constavac* is to drain fluid that accumulates in the wound. This drainage tube will stay in place for approximately 24 hours. The tourniquet is removed and blood once more moves freely through the leg. The knee is wrapped in a bulky bandage that is usually removed the first day after surgery.

The procedure is over. The circulating nurse records the information on the computer, and the surgeons remove their outer clothing layers. The team is winding down.

Fifteen minutes later, Bob R. is being transferred to the recovery room, where close monitoring will be continued. Since he was awake during the entire procedure, he chatted with Dr. K. about fishing and family.

THE POSTANESTHESIA CARE UNIT

Most patients are relaxed and sleepy after transfer to the postanesthesia care unit (PACU) staffed by registered nurses. These RNs are specially trained to provide postoperative care to patients who underwent orthopedic surgery. Some patients suffer from the aftereffects of the anesthesia and feel a bit hung over and nauseous. The body is still encumbered by all kinds of tubes and lines. All surgical patients receive IV fluids to maintain hydration, as well as antibiotics to prevent infections and oxygen. A Foley catheter is inserted into the bladder and drains urine. Some patients may receive a blood transfusion. Finally, patients are still connected to all kinds of monitoring devices with which to check *vital signs* including pulse, heart rate, temperature, blood pressure, and pulmonary pressure. Pain management is initiated (see Chapter 16). Once stabilized, patients are transferred to their in-patient room for the rest of their hospitalization.

YOUR HOSPITAL STAY

(*Note:* This portion is largely adapted from patient literature distributed to patients at the Hospital for Special Surgery. Your hospital may follow a slightly different protocol. See also Chapter 16.)

Once you arrive in your room, you may feel exhausted. The nursing staff will assess and manage your care and assist with activities of daily living (ADLs). At first, there is nothing that you can do for yourself. You can't even turn on your own. You may opt to engage a private-duty nurse or an aide for a day or two, though this is not covered by your insurance.

Rest is an important part of healing, and even though much is going on, relax as much as you can. Nurses will continue to evaluate your health status and vital signs. They are particularly concerned with your blood circulation and temperature. It is normal to have an elevated temperature during the first 72 hours after surgery.

Medications

Make sure that the hospital staff supplies your regular antirheumatic medications (DMARDs, others) as well as other drugs. If not, discuss this matter with nurse or physician. Medications such as methotrexate or Enbrel may be discontinued for days or weeks during and after surgery.

Prevention and Treatment of Circulatory Problems

One of the risk factors after total joint replacement is the formation of thrombi (blood clots) in leg veins as a result of the interrupted blood flow during the operation or because of the forced immobility of the leg. If present, these thrombi may lead to calf pain or leg swelling, or can rarely travel to the lung as a pulmonary embolism.

Anticoagulant therapy is often prescribed to prevent such complications. Commonly prescribed prophylactic drugs include buffered aspirin or Coumadin. The administration of these drugs requires close monitoring by prothrombin time (PT, Protime), a blood test that measures how rapidly your blood is coagulating (clotting).

The exercises shown in Figure 17–3 reduce the risk of circulatory problems specifically associated with total knee replacement. These exercises also strengthen your leg and buttock muscles. During your initial recovery in the hospital, they should be done 10 times, once an hour.[1]

At HSS, the feet are wrapped into a *plexipulse* device. The wrap is attached to a pneumatic compression device that inflates and deflates in a pulse-like fashion, thereby facilitating blood flow through the legs. The plexipulse is usually worn during the first 48 hours after surgery.

Prevention of Lung Problems

Most hospitals provide their patients with a device that helps them breathe deeply to expand their lungs. The inspirometer used at HSS is described in Chapter 16.

---

[1]All the exercises in this chapter (Figs. 17–3, and 17–4), as well as instructions on how to navigate stairs (Fig. 17–5), are taken from *Your Pathway to Recovery: Total Knee Replacement Surgery*, by Suzanne Graziano. Reproduced with the permission of the Department of Nursing Administration, Hospital for Special Surgery.

FIGURE 17-3. Prevention of Circulation Problems. The quad set, gluteal set, and ankle pump exercises are done to improve blood circulation as well as muscle tone. *From* Your Pathway to Recovery, *by Suzanne Graziano, Department of Nursing Administration, HSS.*

To enhance circulation, YOU will be expected to perform these exercises 10 times each, *every hour* while awake.

ANKLE PUMPS: Bend your feet toward you (use your ankles to flex your feet) and away from you (point your feet).

QUAD SETS: Press the backs of your knees into the bed by tightening the front of your thighs. Hold for 6 seconds; relax.

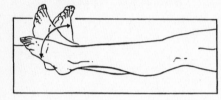 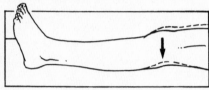

GLUTEAL SETS: Squeeze your buttocks together, causing your hips to be lifted slightly off the bed. Hold for 6 seconds, then release.

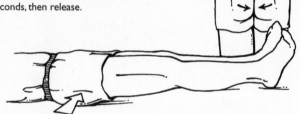

REHABILITATION OF THE KNEE

Passive and Active Exercise

The most crucial part of your recovery concerns the restoration of the mobility of your new knee. Unfortunately, you cannot hold off on rehabilitation until you feel better. It must start immediately. The continuous passive motion (CPM) machine helps to achieve this goal. It continually bends your leg at the knee. A physical therapist will determine the degree of flexion of the knee and the rate at which it is bent. To start, the knee is bent 50° to 60°. The flexion angle is increased gradually to counteract the effects of joint immobilization, enhance the knee's range of motion, and reduce swelling.

Patients differ in their attitude towards the CPM machine. Most patients enjoy the gentle motion the machine supplies; a few dislike it intensely. Nurses and physical therapists recommend that you relax when on the machine. Some surgeons suggest that patients use the machine whenever possible during the day; others limit its use to 4 to 6 hours. While on the machine you can distract yourself by watching television, listening to music, or listening to a book on tape. When off the CPM machine the leg should be kept straight. You can turn the machine on and off. If it becomes too uncomfortable, turn it off when your leg is extended, and, if indicated, call the nurse or the physical therapist.

Passive exercise, as provided by the CPM machine, is insufficient to get your knee into shape. The physical therapist will help with active exercises, and you will participate the day after surgery.

It takes some effort to get out of bed and walk again. The physical therapist will teach you to move to the edge of the bed and sit up with your feet dangling over the side. Then you will stand up, using a walker for assistance and support. You may wonder if your new knee will be able to support you, but the therapist will encourage you to put your full weight on the operated leg as soon as possible. You'll be fine. You may only be able to walk to the door of your room and sit in a chair for a short period of time. Soon you'll walk along the corridors and eat all your meals sitting up in a chair. When you are comfortable navigating with the walker, you'll progress to a cane.

Every surgeon has his or her own set of exercises that the physical therapist will teach you to do at home. The exercises in Figure 17-4 are often added to the exercises in Figure 17–3.

Learning to Do Stairs

Once you are comfortable walking, you will be taught to navigate stairs. The method is clearly outlined in Figure 17–5. If you forget what you were taught, use your head. Walk upstairs with your good leg leading. Walk downstairs with your cane and repaired leg first (during that time the weight is on the unaffected leg), support your weight with a cane, then transfer the weight to the stronger leg.

Pain Management

The first day(s) after surgery, you will experience quite a bit of pain. There is no point braving it. Chapter 16 describes the pain management program used at HSS. The patient-controlled anesthesia (PCA) system

FIGURE 17-4. Additional Commonly Used Exercises After TKR.

From Your Pathway to Recovery, *by Suzanne Graziano, Department of Nursing Administration, HSS.*

Knee flexion
- Sitting on a firm mattress, table or high chair, as shown:
- Bend your operated knee as far back as you can.
- Hold for the count of 6. Relax.
- Perform ___ repetitions, ___ times a day.

(If you are sitting on a mattress, it may be helpful to place a folded towel under your knee.)

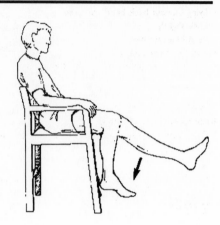

Straight leg raise
- Lying on your back on a firm mattress:
- Keep non-operated leg, hip and knee bent with foot flat on bed.
- Raise straight operated leg until foot is 12" to 15" off bed. Keep knee as straight as possible.
- Hold for the count of 6 and then slowly lower leg to the bed.
- Perform —— repetitions, ___ times a day.

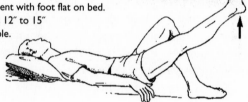

(If you have had operations for both knees, you may have to keep one leg extended as you straight leg raise the other.)

involves a small pump that automatically delivers a small amount of pain medication intravenously or epidurally when needed.

Once the PCA is discontinued, pain can also be controlled by the use of oral medication. Nonpharmacological methods of pain control (relaxation exercises) are also useful.

In addition to these systemic measures, it is important to apply cold packs to your newly operated knee. In the hospital the nursing staff and/or the physical therapists will provide you with cold therapy. You should have cold packs at home in preparation for your return. A large pack of frozen peas is as good as commercial wraps. Make sure that whatever is applied to the surgical area is covered in a towel. The prescribed use of cold therapy is 4 hours per day, 15 to 20 minutes at a time for the first 6 weeks to 2 months after surgery.

FIGURE 17-4. *(continued)*

Hamstring isometrics
• Lying on your back, bend operated
  knee slightly.
• Push heel into bed.
• Hold for the count of 6.
• Perform —— repetitions, ___ times a day.

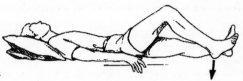

Knee extension while sitting
• From sitting position over side of bed or high chair:

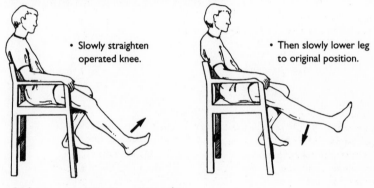

• Slowly straighten
  operated knee.

• Then slowly lower leg
  to original position.

• Perform ___ repetitions, ___ times a day.

Sleeping

Your knee should be extended while you sleep. A rolled towel may be placed under your heel to help you maintain this position. Sometimes the surgeon, nurse, or physical therapist may order a knee splint to ensure that the knee is extended.

Food

You won't be terribly hungry after your surgery, which is just as well. Your bowel will take several days to return to full function; thus, on the day of the surgery your menu only includes ice chips. The next day, you'll be on a clear liquid diet, and on day 3 you'll progress to a full liquid diet, which includes ice cream and soups. On day 4, as you think about going home, it is time for regular food.

FIGURE 17-5. Navigating Stairs After TKR or THR. *From* Your Pathway to Recovery, *by Suzanne Graziano, Department of Nursing Administration, HSS.*

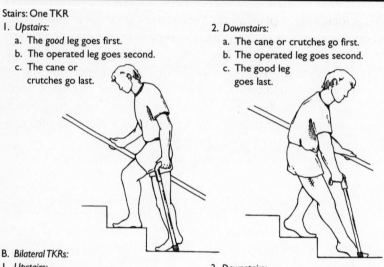

Stairs: One TKR
1. *Upstairs:*
   a. The *good* leg goes first.
   b. The operated leg goes second.
   c. The cane or crutches go last.

2. *Downstairs:*
   a. The cane or crutches go first.
   b. The operated leg goes second.
   c. The good leg goes last.

B. *Bilateral TKRs:*
1. *Upstairs:*
   a. The *stronger* leg goes first.
   b. The *weaker* leg goes second.
   c. The cane or crutches go last.

2. *Downstairs:*
   a. The cane or crutches go first.
   b. The *weaker* leg goes second.
   c. The *stronger* leg goes last.

Personal Hygiene

After the bladder catheter is discontinued (day 1 or 2 after surgery), you are encouraged to get out of bed and use the bathroom. Most likely, you will not have a bowel movement until day 3 or 4 after surgery, and a laxative may be required. Your nurse will assess and manage your progression.

At first, you will be given a sponge bath by the nursing staff, and they will encourage your participation. You will be able to shower once your staples are removed, which is usually 7 to 10 days after surgery.

Activities of Daily Living

In most hospitals the physical therapy staff will suggest activities of daily living devices to help you put on shoes and stockings, or pick up objects from the floor without bending.

Preparing to Go Home

During the 1960s and 1970s, patients used to stay in the hospital for weeks after total joint replacement. Today, most patients are safely discharged on day 4 or 5. It is important to prepare your home before you enter the hospital (see Chapter 16).

Discharge planning is the province of the case manager, and it starts before or as soon as you enter the hospital. Discuss your discharge needs with this health care professional. He or she will evaluate your needs, help you arrange transportation, and recommend a home health care agency if needed. For details, see Chapter 16.

Once you are ready for discharge, make sure that you have:

♦ Your hospital discharge instructions.

♦ Prescriptions and instructions for all newly prescribed medications.

♦ The medications you brought with you to the hospital. (If you gave them to the staff, make sure that they are returned to you.)

♦ Phone numbers of health personnel (physicians, surgeons, physical therapist, case manager) to contact in case of emergency or further clarification of instructions.

♦ Personal items such as dentures, glasses, and hearing aids.

Home and Postsurgery Checkup

Home never looked as good as it does after a hospital stay. Enjoy. Do your exercises and go to bed. You will be tired.

Few doctor visits are as pleasant as those occurring after a successful operation. You may have had a house call from a visiting nurse during the initial recovery period. After 3 to 6 weeks, you will return to see your surgeon. X rays are taken then, and are taken periodically thereafter (after 4 months, and after 1, 2, 5, 10, 15, and 20 years). Most patients can resume driving 6 weeks after surgery.

◆ CHAPTER ◆

18

Surgery of the Hip

This chapter reviews rheumatoid arthritis of the hip and accompanies a patient slated for total hip replacement (THR) to the operating room. Information to protect a new hip during its vulnerable stage is provided.

Total hip replacement (THR) will forever occupy a special place in the annals of surgery. It was the first joint to be successfully replaced, and since the operation reached America's shores during the 1970s, it has enabled millions of otherwise handicapped people to lead pleasurable lives.

People suffering from RA have a hard time deciding which one of their affected joints is the worst. The hip, however, is near the top. There simply is no way of getting away from a badly inflamed hip. It hurts around the clock regardless of whether you are sitting, standing, or lying down.

ANATOMY OF THE HIP

Bony Structure

The hip is the largest joint in the body. It connects the femur, or thighbone, with the pelvis. It is an almost perfect ball-and-socket joint. The ball part is the head of the femur and the socket is the deep cup-like depression of the pelvic bone called the *acetabulum*. As seen in Figure 18–1, the femur divides at its upper end into the *greater trochanter* and the *femoral neck*. The latter terminates in the almost perfectly spherical femoral head.

The hip joint is extremely stable. The acetabulum encloses 40 percent of the head of the femur. Contact is further increased to 50 percent by a layer of dense tissue protruding from both sides of the acetabulum.

Soft Tissues

The principal muscles of the hip include the *flexors* (e.g., the *iliopsoas* muscle), the *extensors* (e.g., the *gluteus maximus*), and the *abductors* (e.g., the *gluteus medius*). You don't have to be a linguist to figure out that the flexors allow the hip to bend, the extensors enable it to straighten, and the abductors allow the thighs to open. Several other muscles enable the hip and leg to rotate and move sideways.

Large nerves innervate the muscles that move a large joint such as the hip. The principal ones include the *sciatic nerve,* the largest nerve of the body, the *femoral nerve,* and the *obturator nerve.*

The sciatic nerve runs from the lumbar region of the spine, down through the pelvis, the buttocks, and the back of the leg. The femoral nerve runs down the front of the thigh, and the obturator runs down the inside of the thigh.

In health the surfaces of the hip joint are covered with cartilage. The entire hip joint is enclosed in a fibrous joint capsule, lined by synovium, which secretes synovial fluid. This synovium is the target of RA, causing it to swell, proliferate, and release large quantitites of immune and inflammatory factors. Eventually, these can destroy the smooth joint surface, causing it to buckle, pit, and develop bone spurs. Before the advent of hip surgery, the hips of patients suffering from advanced RA occasionally fused (grew together).

THE OPERATING ROOM

Frank R. (not his real name) is lying on his side on the operating table. He has elected to be asleep during the surgery, so he is not aware of the bustle that surrounds him. His anesthesiologist, Dr. K., is scrubbing his back with Betadine. Then he carefully locates the right spot for the injection of local anesthetic into the space around the dura mater—the tough membrane surrounding the spinal canal.

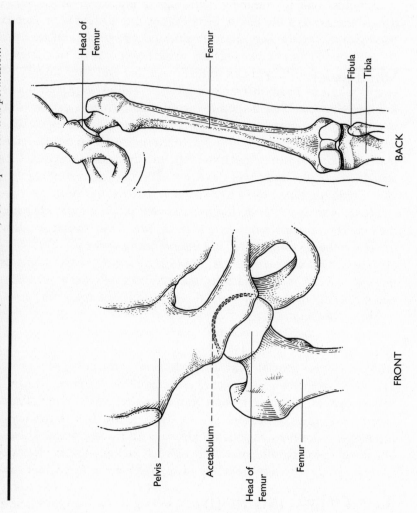

FIGURE 18-1. Anatomy of the Hip. *From* The Columbia Presbyterian Osteoarthritis Handbook, *R. P. Grelsamer and S. Macmillan, 1996. Reproduced with permission.*

Head of Femur

Femur

Fibula

Tibia

BACK

Pelvis

Acetabulum

Head of Femur

Femur

FRONT

"You estimate that the surgery will take no more than 2 hours," he says to Dr. Nestor, and injects the calculated amount of drug.

The surgical team, similar to the one described during TKR surgery, swings into action. One of the two surgical technicians hovers over the instruments, making sure that everything is there. The movable Plexiglas panels are slid into place. The center of the OR is filled with filtered air. The members of the surgical team don their robes and space helmets.

Both of Frank's lower legs are enclosed in elastic stockings. This reduces the risk of blood clot formation during and after surgery. Much care is taken to position Frank properly. A pillow is placed under his side, another between his legs. A large plastic sheet separates Frank's upper body and the anesthesiologist from his trunk and legs.

The leg is scrubbed with a powerful antiseptic, then it is covered with a plastic sheet lined with specially treated antiseptic gauze. Except for the operative field, Frank disappears under billows of sterile blue sheets. Tubing and electric leads connect him to various instruments. A solution containing antibiotics slowly drips into the veins of his arm. As the operation proceeds, Dr. K. calls for a unit of blood, which is administered intravenously. Oxygen slowly enters Frank's nose. This will help oxygenate his blood and reduce trauma. Dr. Nestor looks at Frank's X rays, prominently displayed on a light box, asks for a sterile marking pen, and marks the incision.

DESIGN OF THE TOTAL HIP

The artificial hip implants used today (Fig. 18-2) are basically the same as those developed by Dr. John Charnley in Brighton, England, during the 1960s (for details, see Chapter 16), although they are somewhat modified. Charnley's femoral component was all in one piece. Today, the head of the femur is a separate little ball that gets impacted onto the stem. Charnley's cup consisted entirely of high-density polyethylene. Today, the cup is made from a metal alloy lined with a thick layer of polyethylene. Dr. Nestor also uses a slightly different surgical approach to reach the hip, which interferes less with the muscle and nerve tissue.

The biggest change, however, concerns the cement. The major and most common problem with implants has always been loosening. The reason for this phenomenon has never quite been established. One more recent hypothesis attributes it to the microscopic particles resulting from the wearing down of the prosthesis, especially of its polymer component.

FIGURE 18-2. Total Hip Prostheses.

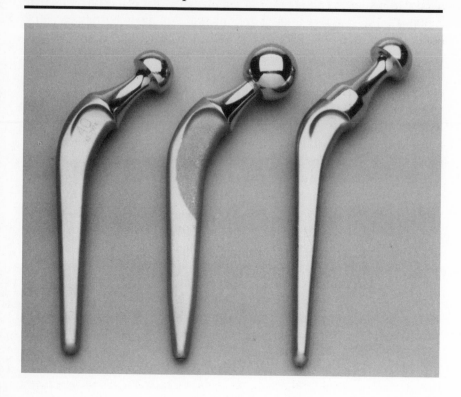

Cementless prostheses are nothing new. Implants, whose surface is porous to permit the in-growth of bone, have been available for some time. Dr. Nestor and other surgeons also routinely insert the cup portion of the prothesis into the pelvic bone, where in-growth and the fibrous tissue will keep it in place.

The choice of whether to cement the hip, however, is made individually for each patient. Dr. Nestor is more inclined to use cemented hips for older patients such as Frank.

BACK TO THE OPERATING ROOM

Dr. Nestor uses a scalpel to cut through the skin and muscle tissue. He separates the various layers of muscle and fat tissue until he reaches the hip joint. The synovium is overgrown and the surfaces of the bones are full of pits and small craters. The surgeon rapidly cuts off its diseased head. He passes it to the surgical technician, who places it in a small container. The pathology laboratory at HSS will examine this piece of bone in great detail. Then Dr. Nestor turns his attention to the acetabulum. It is carefully cleaned and shaved down with a rounded circular drill called an acetabular reamer. He uses increasingly large drill heads, until the cavity is smooth and clean. Because of the hip's central location, blood flow cannot be interrupted, and there is some blood loss. Assistants using vacuum suction keep the site of the operation free of bone chips, blood, and other debris. From time to time, they wash the site with saline solution.

The circulating nurse obtains the appropriate implant size from inventory. She double-checks the size and identification numbers on the boxes with the surgical technician. The implant is unwrapped and passed to the surgical team. The acetabular components, consisting of a metal shell and a liner made from ultrahigh-density polyethylene, is inserted in the prepared cavity.

Returning to the femur, Dr. Nestor prepares the femoral canal so that it can receive the long stem of the femoral component. The alignment of the femur and acetabulum is checked with a trial femoral component, which is slid into the femoral canal. The surgical team carefully evaluates how the hip and leg move, and whether the length of the operated leg will match the length of the other. Once everybody is satisfied, the team is ready to insert and cement the femoral stem. The circulating nurse obtains the appropriate size, three units of cement powder, and three units of mixer.

The powder and mixer are poured into a coffee mill–type machine that is really a miniature cement mixer. The OR fills with the familiar odor of freshly mixed epoxy glue. The mixed cement is put into a syringe and handed to the surgical team, who inject it into the femoral canal. Then the stem of the prosthesis is slid into the canal and hammered into place. Finally, the surgeon impacts the separate femoral head onto the stem.

The surgeon carefully inspects the cavity, making sure that it is free of debris. Frank's leg is bent, straightened, and twisted. Everything seems to be in ship-shape order and it's time to close the wound. As in the case of the knee, a thin plastic tube is left in place. It will drain fluid from the wound for approximately 24 hours. Slowly, layer by layer, muscle tissue and skin layers are returned to their place and stitched back together. When this is done, Dr. Nestor goes to the waiting room to tell Frank's wife that the operation is successfully concluded.

YOUR HOSPITAL STAY

(*Note:* The following is based on the routine used at the Hospital for Special Surgery as described in their patient literature. Your hospital may follow a slightly different protocol or guideline. See also Chapters 16 and 17.)

Frank continues to sleep in the recovery room and is unaware of the monitoring and even of the additional pint of blood he receives. He finally wakes up in his own room, feeling dazed, sore, and sleepy. He discovers that his leg is suspended in an abating sling. A trapeze device hangs down from the bed's rail. Later, he will use it to raise himself up in bed. A heavy dressing covers the surgical site.

Even though he feels uncomfortable and is a bit nauseous, Frank appreciates that his hip feels distinctly better. The nagging, burning pain that had increasingly plagued him through the years is gone.

Frank meets Daisy, one of two private-duty nurses who are to care for him for 48 hours. They will assess him and provide the necessary care during this initial healing process. Catheters and lines still emerge from his body. A thin cannula to his nose still delivers extra oxygen. The oxygen therapy is essential for the cardiovascular system during the initial healing time. An IV line continues to provide the body with fluid and prophylactic antibiotics, and allows easy access for the administration of other medications (analgesics, others) should they be needed. A Foley catheter empties the bladder.

Within 24 to 48 hours, the catheters and lines (bladder catheter, IV drip, tube draining the wound) are usually discontinued and your body regains its independence. By day 1 after surgery, the surgical dressing will be gone. Your leg, which might have felt like a separate entity, again feels as if it is yours.

Food progresses from ice chips (day of the surgery) to clear liquids to a full liquid diet and/or soft foods. By day 3, you are back on a regular hospital diet.

Pain Management

Pain is present after every surgical procedure. Most hospitals make a great effort to alleviate postsurgical pain. The patient-controlled anesthesia (PCA) used at HSS was described in detail in Chapter 16. Other hospitals may control pain by intravenous injection of strong analgesics or medication taken by mouth. You will only use strong analgesics during the first day(s) after surgery, then you will switch to milder analgesics. Other ways of controlling pain include the application of cold packs and the relaxation exercises described in Chapter 14. Since it is important to exercise in spite of your pain, it is advisable to take pain medication prior to your exercise session. Make sure that the hospital staff supplies your regular antirheumatic medications (DMARDs, others) as well as other drugs you take regularly. If there is a problem, discuss it with a nurse or physician. Methotrexate or Enbrel are sometimes halted the week of the surgery and thereafter.

Prevention and Treatment of Circulatory Problems

Most hospitals provide their patients with a device that helps them breathe deeply to prevent pulmonary complications. The inspirometer used at HSS is described in Chapter 16 and its use is illustrated in Figure 16–2.

To improve your circulation, you will be asked to do ankle pumps, quad and gluteal sets (see Fig. 17–3) 10 times every hour while awake. These exercises will also improve blood circulation and muscle tone.

In addition to these conservative measures, your physician may decide that you should receive anticoagulant therapy (medication preventing blood clot formation). (For details, see Chapter 17.)

Personal Hygiene

Your bowels, which you cleaned out so conscientiously before surgery, are reluctant to start functioning again. At HSS, laxatives are usually given on the third day after surgery. It is important to remember that you should not crouch down on a toilet seat. In the hospital you will have a high toilet or a high commode.

You will wash as best as you can with a sponge or washcloth. You can shower—preferably in a stall shower—when your staples have been removed.

PROTECTING YOUR NEW HIP[1]

Your new hip will feel so good that you may tend to overuse it. It will, however, take months for your new hip to heal and anchor to its

[1]The information in this section, as well as the accompanying table and illustrations, are taken with permission from the manual Suzanne Graziano, RN, MS, ONC, CAN, Clinical Nurse Specialist, has written for the Patient Education Course, which was developed under the aegis of the Department of Nursing Administration at HSS.

surroundings. If you move it beyond its limits too soon, it may dislocate. During the healing period, the new hip must be protected. The guidelines used at HSS for the protection of a freshly operated hip are presented in Table 18–1. Figures 18–3 to 18–6 amplify these instructions. Precautions to be taken during sexual intercourse are illustrated in Figure 18–7. The precautions recommended by the HSS are universal. Your surgeon will tell you when they can be disregarded.

TABLE 18-1. Precaution Guidelines for Total Hip Replacement

1. Do not bend your hip more than 90° by lifting your knee, by bending over at your waist, or by squatting down.

2. Do not cross your legs or ankles when lying, standing, or sitting.

3. Avoid sitting on low, soft chairs, such as sofas, easy chairs, etc. You must sit on a firm chair (preferably with arms) using two firm pillows to raise the height of the seat. (It is important to plan for appropriate seating around your house before you go to the hospital.) Also, your bed must be at least 18 inches high. When you sit on the bed your knee must be lower than your hip joint (see Fig. 18–3). If necessary, add another mattress to raise your bed to the proper height.

4. When entering or traveling by car:

   a. Sit in the front passenger seat on two pillows.

   b. Make sure that the car seat is slid all the way back before entering.

   c. Enter from the street level rather than the curb in order to avoid bending your hip.

   d. Sit down with your buttocks first, then swing your legs around.

5. Do not allow your knees to come together when sitting or lying in bed. Keep your knees well apart at all times. When lying on your unaffected side, keep two pillows between your legs.

6. Use a raised toilet seat.

7. Do not take a tub bath yet. You may shower after your sutures are out. A walk-in shower is preferable. (Your surgeon will let you know when you may start taking a bath.) If your shower is in a bath, enter with your good leg. Do not bend your operated leg more than 90°.

8. Do not resume driving until you have your surgeon's permission.

9. During intercourse follow the precautions outlined in Figure 18–7.

Source: From *Your Pathway to Recovery, Total Hip Replacement Surgery,* by Suzanne Graziano. Reproduced with the permission of the Department of Nursing Administration, Hospital for Special Surgery.

FIGURE 18-3. How to Sleep After THR. *From* Your Pathway to Recovery, *by Suzanne Graziano, Department of Nursing Administration, HSS.*

Bed positioning
* Try to keep kneecaps pointed towards the ceiling.
* Use the slings to sleep in while you are in the hospital.
* The head of your bed should be no more than half upright (45°).
* When exercising or getting out of bed, the bed should be flat.

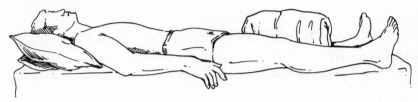

When lying on your back, keep a folded pillow between your knees.

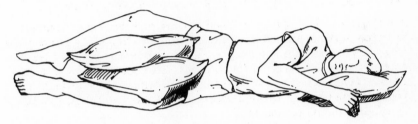

When lying on your unoperated side, place two pillows between your legs.

* DO NOT LIE ON YOUR OPERATED SIDE!

Sleeping

You can sleep on your nonoperated side or on your back. When lying on your side, keep two pillows between your legs to prevent them from closing (see Table 18–1 and Figure 18–3). Patients who underwent a bilateral (both sides) THR must sleep on their back.

Remember the instructions detailed in Table 18–1 at all times. The illustrations provided in Figures 18–3 to 18–6 should be reviewed.

Dressing

Because you may not bend your hip more than 90°, you will have a tough time putting on shoes and socks. Use a stocking aid to put on and take off stockings. You must use the stocking aid for your nonoperated leg, too. Use a long shoehorn to put on shoes. Women should not wear pantyhose for months after surgery because putting them on and off

FIGURE 18-4. Sitting

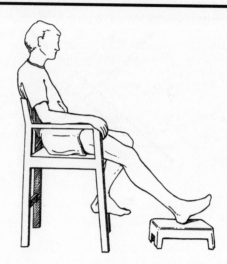

When sitting

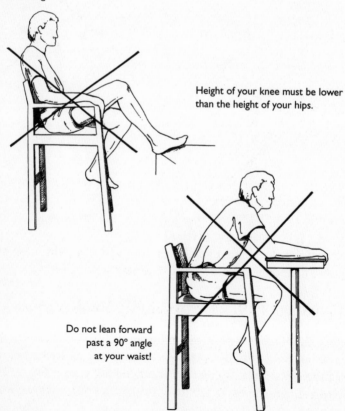

Height of your knee must be lower than the height of your hips.

Do not lean forward past a 90° angle at your waist!

FIGURE 18-5. Positioning

Do not cross your legs when lying, sitting, or standing.

Do not roll legs inwards towards each other.
Your feet should be pointed up towards ceiling
or outward.

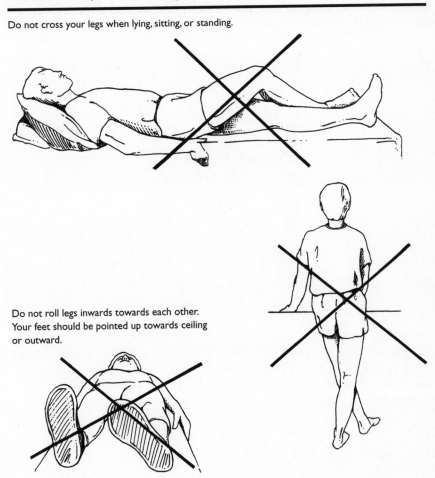

pushes the knees together. Long stockings held up by a garter belt are
okay, but socks, including knee-highs, are more comfortable.

Sexual Intercourse Following Total Hip Replacement

The majority of patients will enjoy resuming sexual intercourse after hip
replacement. As a matter of fact, such intimacy may be particularly enjoyable now that the constant, nagging pain has been alleviated. In general,
most people can resume intercourse 4 to 6 weeks after surgery, when the

FIGURE 18-6. Dressing

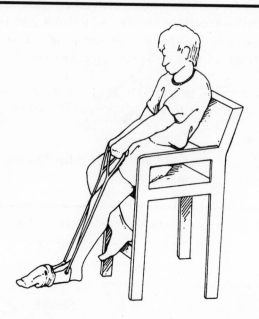

incision site and muscles around the hip joint have healed. Initially, however, your new hip must be protected from excessive flexion, abduction, and internal rotation. Suzanne Graziano and her team have provided you with an illustration on how to resume an enjoyable sex life (Fig. 18-7).

REHABILITATION

Exercises after THR

Every surgeon has his or her specific rehabilitation program to be implemented by your physical therapist. The following is a review of the exercises most commonly used.

As compared to TKR patients, THR patients are fortunate. There is no continuous passive motion machine. Instead, the most important exercise for the hip is walking, which everybody knows how to do. However, it will take you some time until you are able to walk freely.

You will have to learn to sit up, stand, and gain enough confidence in your new hip to use it. Most patients achieve this goal within the 5 days of their hospital stay.

A physical therapist will be present when you first sit up. To sit and stand, you have to sidle to the edge of your bed. This, at first, is a major undertaking, because you are not allowed to bend your hip. Once at the edge of the bed, it is simple to turn and let your feet dangle. Always sit for a minute at the edge of the bed to give your blood pressure time to equalize.

The physical therapist will be at your side when you first stand. In addition, you will hold on to a walker. You will be told how much weight

FIGURE 18-7. **Protecting Your New Hip During Sexual Intercourse.** *From* Your Pathway to Recovery, *by Suzanne Graziano, Department of Nursing Administration, HSS.*

Positions for Intercourse which *Do Conform* to Precautions of Total Hip Replacement

Pillows can be used under the knees, back, and/or side for comfort and support.

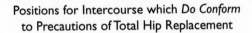

Patient on the bottom: partner on the top.

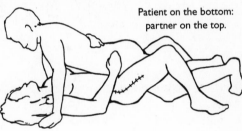

Patient on the top: partner on the bottom.

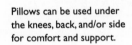

Standing position for both the patient and partner.

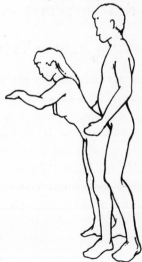

Patient lying on side with operated leg on top.

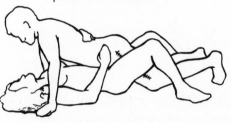

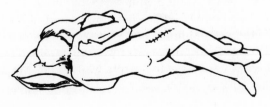

FIGURE 18-7. *(continued)*

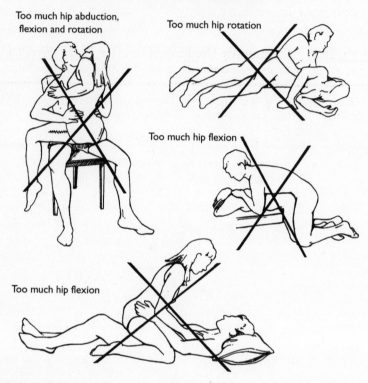

Positions for Intercourse *To Be Avoided*
Following Total Hip Replacement

Too much hip abduction, flexion and rotation

Too much hip rotation

Too much hip flexion

Too much hip flexion

Obviously, there are other safe and unsafe positions and methods of obtaining sexual satisfaction. Please think them through. If necessary, please be ready to try something new to help protect your new hip(s).

to put on your new hip (this varies from 20 percent to weight bearing as tolerated). Though this sounds confusing, the staff will coach you through. Your new hip will not collapse when you stand. Taking a few steps is all you have to do the first day, especially since you are busy pumping your ankles, squeezing your buttocks, and inhaling with the inspirometer.

The routine will be repeated the next day: getting out of bed, walking a short distance with the help of the nurse or the physical therapist, sitting in the comfortably high hip chair for periods of up to 30 minutes. By now, you should feel almost human and you will start to enjoy your new hip. By the third day after surgery, when you feel really comfortable with your walker, depending on your weight-bearing status, you may be switched to a cane.

While in the hospital you will continue to practice getting in and out of bed, sitting in a chair, and walking up and down the corridors. Your physical therapist will discuss your home exercise program with you. Commonly used exercises are shown in Figure 18–8.

FIGURE 18-8. Commonly Used Exercises after THR. *From* Your Pathway to Recovery, *by Suzanne Graziano, Department of Nursing Administration, HSS.*

On back
1. Quad sets
   a. Tighten both knee muscles by pressing knees down into bed.
   b. Hold for count of 6.
   c. Relax.
   d. Perform ___ repetitions, ___ times a day.

2. Gluteal sets
   a. Pinch buttocks together.
   b. Hold for count of 6.
   c. Relax.
   d. Perform ___ repetitions, ___ times a day.

3. Ankle circles (not shown)
   a. Keeping legs flat on bed, make circles with your ankles.
   b. Perform ___ repetitions, ___ times a day.

4. Internal rotation to neutral
   a. Roll operated leg inwards so that your kneecap and foot are pointed towards the ceiling.
   b. Perform ___ repetitions, ___ times a day.

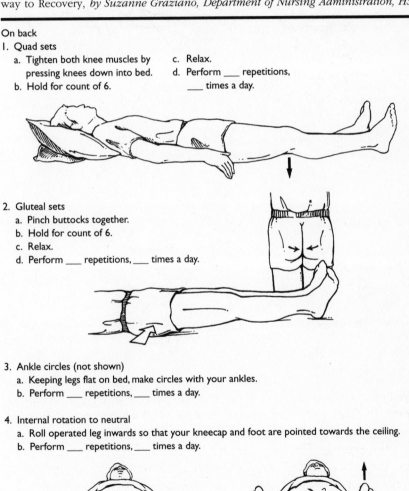

FIGURE 18-8. *(continued)*

5. Lying on back
   a. Bend hip and knee of operated side to about 40°–45°.
   b. Hold for 6 seconds.
   c. Slowly lower your leg and relax.
   d. Perform ___ repetitions, ___ times a day.

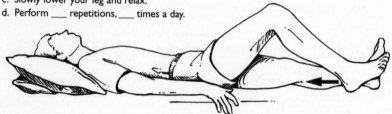

6. Lying on back
   Pillow between legs. Bend unoperated leg with foot flat on bed.
   a. Raise operated leg, keeping it straight, to height of pillow.
   b. Lower leg slowly—keeping knee straight.
   c. Perform ___ repetitions, ___ times a day.
   d. NOTE: If you experience any pain in the groin, hold off on this exercise for now. Try again 3–7 days later. If you still experience pain, delay trying it again.

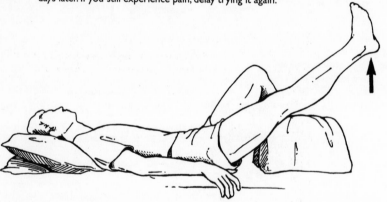

FIGURE 18-8. *(continued)*

Sitting

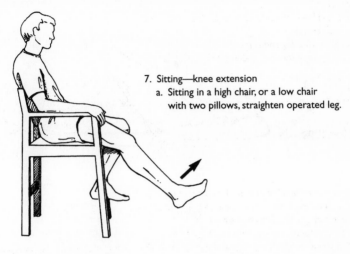

7. Sitting—knee extension
   a. Sitting in a high chair, or a low chair
      with two pillows, straighten operated leg.

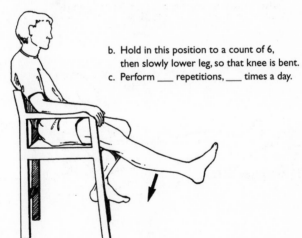

   b. Hold in this position to a count of 6,
      then slowly lower leg, so that knee is bent.
   c. Perform ___ repetitions, ___ times a day.

FIGURE 18-8. *(continued)*

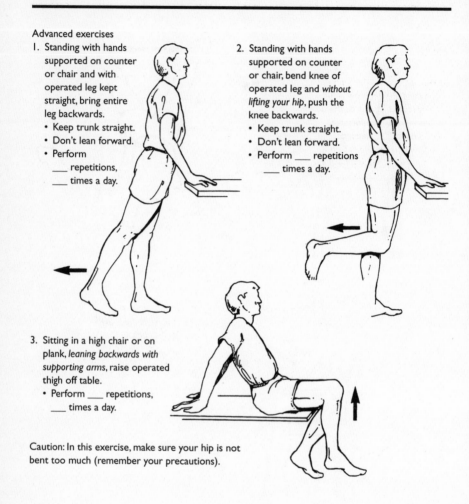

Advanced exercises

1. Standing with hands supported on counter or chair and with operated leg kept straight, bring entire leg backwards.
   - Keep trunk straight.
   - Don't lean forward.
   - Perform ___ repetitions, ___ times a day.

2. Standing with hands supported on counter or chair, bend knee of operated leg and *without lifting your hip*, push the knee backwards.
   - Keep trunk straight.
   - Don't lean forward.
   - Perform ___ repetitions ___ times a day.

3. Sitting in a high chair or on plank, *leaning backwards with supporting arms*, raise operated thigh off table.
   - Perform ___ repetitions, ___ times a day.

Caution: In this exercise, make sure your hip is not bent too much (remember your precautions).

FIGURE 18-8. *(continued)*

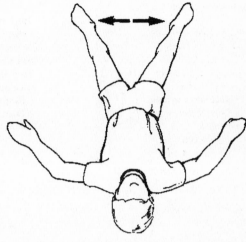

4. Hip Abduction—lying on back
   • Lifting slightly, move your operated leg out to the side as far as is comfortable.
   • Hold for ___ seconds.
   • Slowly relax and return it to neutral, relaxed position.
   • Perform ___ repetitions, ___ times a day.

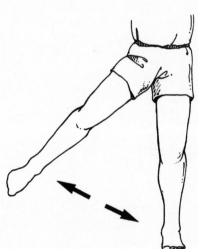

5. Hip Abduction—standing
   • Stand, holding on to a solid object for balance.
   • Bring operated leg out to side, without letting it come forward.
   • Hold for ___ seconds, then slowly relax.
   • Perform ___ repetitions, ___ times a day.

PREPARING TO GO HOME

Since you need to follow the total hip replacement precautions (see Table 18–1), you may need some special gadgets, especially if you live alone. These include:

◆ A portable raised toilet seat (essential)

◆ A contraption to put on your stockings (see Fig. 18–6) and a long-handled shoehorn for putting on shoes

◆ A long-handled pair of pincers that enables you to pick up items from the floor

◆ A high chair with arms

Hopefully, you have procured these items before your surgery. A therapist or the nursing staff will teach you how to use these gadgets. You will also be taught to climb stairs. For details, see Figure 17-5. Even though you can elevate the seat of an ordinary chair with two hard pillows, the sturdy hip chairs with arm rests are good to have. The chairs can often be rented from a surgical supply company.

DISCHARGE

As previously discussed, make sure that you have:

◆ The hospital discharge papers.

◆ Prescriptions and instructions for all newly prescribed medications.

◆ The medications you brought with you to the hospital. (If you gave them to the staff, make sure that they are returned to you.)

◆ Phone numbers of health personnel (physicians, surgeons, physical therapist, and case manager) to contact in case of emergency.

◆ Your dentures, glasses, and hearing aid.

◆ Information on how, when, and where to get blood tests to monitor your blood coagulation if you are taking Coumadin, and, if necessary, which doctor will adjust the dosage.

HOME

You will be happy to be home, though you are still extremely frail and tired. You will do very little in addition to your prescribed exercises, which in the beginning consist mostly of walking. You will sleep a lot in your elevated bed. It usually takes 6 to 8 weeks until you are allowed to close your legs and flex your leg above 90°.

Ten days after surgery, you may be visited at home by a nurse. After 3–6 weeks, you'll return to the doctor for X rays and a physical. Prophylactic measures such as wearing elastic stockings and using a raised toilet seat will be discontinued after 6 weeks, when you'll also be allowed to start driving. Many surgeons ask their patients to return after 4 months. Routine X rays are taken after 1, 2, 5, 10, 15, and 20 years.

◆ CHAPTER ◆

19

The Upper Extremities and the Feet

This chapter reviews the surgical repair of the hand. Rheumatoid arthritis and surgery of the elbows, shoulders, and feet are also discussed. (See Chapter 13 for anatomy and RA of the hand, joint protection, and therapy.)

SURGICAL REPAIR OF THE RHEUMATOID HAND

Modern reconstructive hand surgery dates from the 1960s. Before that time, hand surgery for RA simply consisted of exposing the finger joints and repairing them by removing the inflamed synovium, removing other extraneous tissue, and repositioning or reconnecting the tendons. Such arthroplasties were only moderately successful, mostly because they did not restore the joint space that is crucial to the smooth working of any joint. By the 1960s, several surgeons had already developed hinged implants fashioned out of metal, but as in the case of the knee, these prostheses loosened quickly and did not work very well.

At about that time, Alfred B. Swanson, who spent almost his entire professional career at Blodget Memorial Hospital in Grand Rapids, Michigan, started to investigate the use of medical-grade synthetic polymers.

Silicone rubber—a synthetic polymer first developed in the 1930s—seemed ideal. Extensive animal experimentation showed that the material was tolerated by living tissue. Like ordinary rubber, to which it is closely related, the hardness of silicone rubber can be modified by using various additives.

At first, Swanson used silicone rubber implants for lower extremity amputees. These were well tolerated, and Swanson considered using the material in hand surgery. The surgeon embarked on a yearlong study of suitable implants for the hands.

The joints of the finger are different from those encountered elsewhere in the body. They are extremely small and very mobile. The principal function of a finger implant is:

◆ To create or preserve an appropriate joint space

◆ To provide the finger with stability so that it maintains its proper alignment

◆ To maintain its elasticity during flexion

In 1963, Swanson started to use silicone rubber implants. The surgeon simply preserved the joint space by inserting a hand-carved silicone sponge in the metacarpal-phalangeal joint (MCP) during arthroplasty. The results were good, but this interpositional material could not maintain joint alignment and stability. Swanson describes the development of the prostheses in his book, *Flexible Implant Resection Arthroplasty in the Hand and Extremities* (C.V. Mosby, 1973): "We hand-carved a double-stemmed silicone implant that could bridge the joint space to provide some degree of stability and at the same time allow articular motion through the intrinsic flex qualities of the material."

Though results were promising, much work needed to be done. Swanson tested a variety of shapes, for instance, changing the exact configuration and height of the ridge separating the two arrow-shaped extensions of the prosthesis. He modified the hardness of the silicone rubber and developed a machine in which to flex-test his implants. The final version of the implant endured more than 600 million flexion-extension movements without any change. The final model—called the *distributing-load flexible hinge*—is available in nine different sizes (Fig. 19-1). The operation during which these prostheses are implanted is called *flexible implant arthroplasty of the fingers*. The little wedge-shaped objects look so simple that it is hard to recognize the extent to which they have revolutionized hand surgery.

FIGURE 19-1. Swanson Implant. This small Swanson finger joint implant, with protective titanium grommets, designed by Alfred R. Swanson, has revolutionized hand surgery. Dr. Swanson also developed various other silicone rubber implants including ones for the elbow, wrist, trapezius, great toe, radial and ulnar heads. *Photo courtesy of Wright Medical Technology, Inc.*

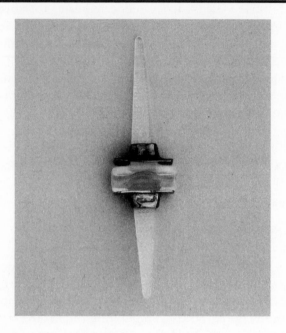

Dr. Swanson also developed various other silicone rubber implants including ones for the elbow, wrist, trapezius, great toe, radial and ulnar heads.

The results of few surgical procedures are as cosmetically pleasing as hand surgery. Rheumatologists and hand surgeons are aware that the cosmetic results of hand surgery can impact positively on the way patients feel about themselves. Functional improvement, however, is variable, and hand deformities can recur after reconstruction.

Hand surgery is always carried out under regional anesthesia (see Chapter 16). Care is taken to halt blood flow into the limb temporarily so that the surgeon can operate in a bloodless field. This is achieved by pushing the blood of the arm into the general circulation and placing a tourniquet around the upper arm. Blood flow can be safely interrupted for 2 hours.

During surgery the joint is exposed. If necessary, the surgeon removes the head of the affected phalanges. The canals of the adjoining phalanges are reamed out. A test implant is inserted to check the appropriate fit before the permanent implant is slipped into the canals. Rheumatoid arthritis often plays havoc with the tendons and ligaments of the hand. These are repaired and repositioned during surgery. The human hand fortunately contains a few less-essential tendons that can be used as spares during the reconstructive process. Before closing the wound, the surgeon tests how well the repaired hand opens and closes. Then the surgeon washes the entire surgical site with anticlotting solution. The wound is dressed and the entire hand is carefully positioned for healing.

As opposed to hips and knees, which can be used soon after surgery, hands heal slowly. As Swanson stated, "The greatest challenge in the postoperative rehabilitation of finger-joint arthroplasty is to maintain the proper balance between good healing...and the desired tension... to obtain the desired range of motion."

After 5 to 7 days, the patient is fitted with a splint (Fig. 19-2) by a hand therapist, who supervises the rehabilitation from then on. After flexible implant arthroplasty, the fingers are suspended in a dynamic

FIGURE 19-2. A Dynamic Hand Splint. A dynamic brace provides the wrist with stability. Finger slings hanging from a cross bar lift up the operated-on joints and prevent ulnar deviation by pulling from the radial side. A system of rubber bands maintains the repaired fingers in their appropriate position. Most often fingers are flexed at an angle of 70°. *Illustration courtesy of Annabel Griffith, Hospital for Special Surgery.*

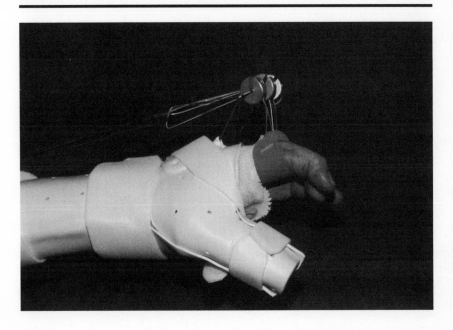

space-age–looking brace that becomes the mainstay of the therapy for the next 6 weeks or so.

At first, the splint is only removed when performing the rigorously prescribed exercises. After about 6 weeks, the splint is only worn at night. The surgeon and hand therapist provide the patient with a home exercise program. Hand exercises are highly individualized. Figure 19-3 illustrates the results of hand surgery.

RA AND SURGICAL REPAIR OF THE RHEUMATOID WRIST

The anatomy of the wrist has been discussed in Chapter 13 as part of the anatomy of the hand. Rheumatoid arthritis often affects the wrist. It is so closely associated with the hand that the two are usually treated together by hand therapists. Some of the routine hand exercises strengthen the wrist. Most of the prescribed splints support the wrist as a matter of course.

Carpal tunnel syndrome occurs frequently in patients suffering from RA. The median nerve that transmits messages to and from the thumb, index, long, and ring fingers, passes through a ligamentous passage or tunnel. During certain conditions (RA, pregnancy, repetitive motions such as computer inputting and knitting) the tissues surrounding this tunnel may swell and compress these nerves, causing numbness, swelling, and eventually pain. Later symptoms may cause muscle wasting.

The condition is most commonly treated with anti-inflammatory drugs and splinting, often only at night, or cortisone injections. If necessary, carpal tunnel syndrome may require surgical decompression of the tunnel, thereby releasing the median nerve.

Surgical treatment of the wrist may involve a synovectomy (removal of the inflamed joint tissues), removal of bone, or total fusion of the carpal bones (arthroplasty). Surgery is also indicated when the inflammation and swelling of the wrist persists and threatens to rupture the large extensor tendons of the hand. A fused wrist is painless, extremely stable, and quite functional.

RA AND SURGICAL REPAIR OF THE RHEUMATOID ELBOW

The elbow corresponds to the knee. It is essential to the movement of the arm and the hand. It allows the hand to move around the body—for

FIGURE 19-3. Results of Hand Surgery. Arthritic hands before and after surgical reconstruction of the knuckles using implants designed by Alfred B. Swanson. The surgery has been used successfully in hundreds of thousands of cases worldwide since 1969. Although this technique will not fully restore the joints to normal, it can relieve pain and improve function. *Photo courtesy of Wright Medical Technology, Inc.*

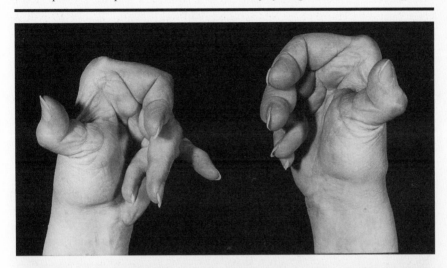

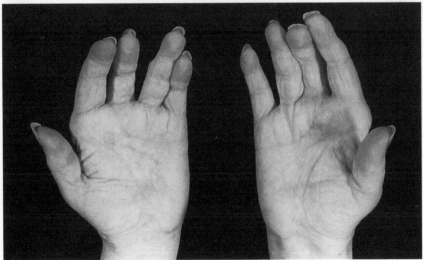

instance, enabling it to bring food to the mouth. The elbow can also twist and turn, permitting the lower arm to move independently of the shoulder.

The elbow is the meeting place of three bones: the humerus or upper arm bone; the ulna, which is the longer and thicker of the two forearm bones; and the radius, which is the thinner one. The elbow joint is really two joints in one. The principal elbow joint, connecting the humerus and the ulna, is a hinge. The second joint, which connects the head of the radius to the ulna, is responsible for the twisting motion. Both joints are enclosed in a single joint cavity.

The poorly protected elbow joint relies on a complex network of muscles, tendons, and ligaments, all cushioned by the small fluid-filled pouches called bursae. These structures can become inflamed. You may be familiar with the tendinitis commonly referred as tennis elbow.

RA of the elbow is common. As the disease progresses, there is destruction of the articular cartilage, joint space narrowing, impairment of the soft tissues, and bone loss. As expected, these lead to pain, loss of function, and instability. Initially, the condition is treated with anti-inflammatory drugs, rest, heat, ice, and/or cortisone injections. A hinged splint, usually worn only at night, may prove helpful. As always, it is important to avoid stressing the joint by having heavy objects (groceries, handbags, and briefcases) dangle from the end of the arm (see Chapter 13).

The elbow is difficult to fix because it is very exposed and poorly protected by soft tissues. As with other joints, surgery of the elbow progresses from a simple synovectomy (removal of the inflamed lining of the joint capsule) to repair, arthrodesis (fusion), or total replacement.

During resection arthoplasty, the elbow is repaired by using the existing tissues. The surgery relieves pain in 80 percent of all patients, but the functional results leave much to be desired. Somewhat better results are achieved by interposition arthroplasty. In order to preserve as much of the normal joint structure, less bone is removed and the surfaces of the joint are lined with either biological or synthetic material. According to Dr. Bryan Nestor, results of this type of surgery are only fair. Arthrodesis of the elbow is used as a last resort, because a rigid elbow is extremely debilitating.

It is thus gratifying that at long last surgeons have come up with a total elbow. Two types of prostheses are available. One type is semi-constrained—that is, the ulnar (lower bone of the arm) and humoral (upper bone of the arm) parts are loosely connected. The other is unrestrained, in which the two halves of the prosthesis are totally separated. As expected, there is an increased risk of loosening with the semiconstrained prosthesis and an increased tendency to instability with the unrestained model. Rehabilitation exercises begin soon after surgery. Some surgeons advocate a continuous passive motion machine similar to the one used during knee surgery. Only 1 to 2 pounds may be lifted with the operated arm during the first 2 months; a maximum limit of 5 to 10 pounds is imposed thereafter. As compared with other joints, the infection risk of total elbow replacement is relatively high—a complication that seems to be related to the vulnerable anatomical position of the elbow. Experience, improvement in the surgical technique used, and routine use of antibiotics is reducing the incidence.

Results with the total elbow replacement are good. Some pain relief and much improved function occur in over 90 percent of patients.

RA AND SURGICAL REPAIR OF THE RHEUMATOID SHOULDER

The three bones that comprise the shoulder are the upper arm bone (humerus), the shoulder blade (scapula), and the collarbone or clavicle. It is easy to feel these bones. The upper edge of the shoulder blade sticks out in the back; the head of the humerus is the nice, round shape that we call the shoulder; and the clavicle is the long, thin bone that runs from the base of the neck to the shoulder (Fig. 19-4).

A conglomerate of four joints connects these bones, sometimes collectively referred to as the *shoulder girdle*. The main shoulder joint is the *glenohumeral joint* that connects the head of the humerus with the shoulder blade. This joint is a ball-and-socket joint like the hip. The shoulder socket (glenoid fossa), however, is much shallower than the acetabulum, and shoulders frequently dislocate.

Rheumatoid arthritis frequently affects the shoulder. A careful evaluation is essential to determine whether the pain is caused by articular (comes from the joint) degeneration or damage to the soft tissues. Shoulder pain can also originate in the cervical spine. Shoulder pain is treated with anti-inflammatory drugs, rest, and cortisone injections. Rest may involve supporting the arm in a sling.

Since the shoulder is so mobile, exercises are particularly important. As always, your physician should prescribe these exercises. Specific exercises for the shoulder are illustrated in Chapter 12.

Shoulder surgery may involve repair of the many muscles, tendons, and ligaments that "work" the shoulder. Tears often occur in the rotator cuff—a series of ligaments and tendons that form a perfect envelope around the glenohumeral joint. In view of the fact that the shoulder is exposed and poorly protected by muscle tissue, surgical repair of the shoulder joint is difficult.

Much progress has been made in the development of a total shoulder prosthesis. Actually, Dr. Charles Neer II had developed a prosthesis that replaced the head of the humerus at Columbia Presbyterian Medical

FIGURE 19-4. Anatomy of the Shoulder. The shoulder is an extremely mobile joint. *From* The Columbia Presbyterian Osteoarthritis Handbook, *R. P. Grelsamer and S. Loebl, eds. Macmillan, 1996. Reproduced with permission.*

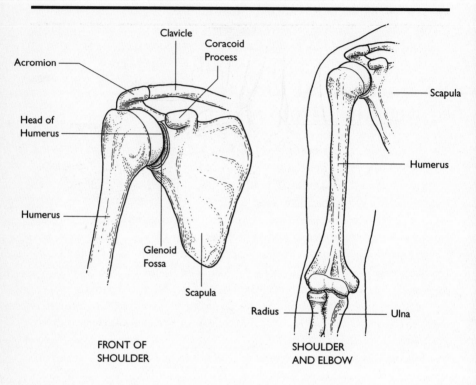

Center in 1951. This prosthesis consisted of an umbrella-shaped head attached to a metal stem. The "umbrella" replaced the head of the humerus, and the stem fitted into the femoral canal. This half prosthesis was quite successful. A total shoulder, in which the head of the humerus is replaced by a metal alloy ball and a synthetic polymer liner, is used for the glenoid fossa, followed the development of the total hip.

RA AND SURGICAL REPAIR OF THE RHEUMATOID FOOT

The human foot resembles the hand. It consists of 26 bones arranged in the hindfoot, the midfoot, and the forefoot (Fig. 19-5). The hindfoot consists of two bones: the *calcaneus,* or heel bone, and the *talus,* or ankle

FIGURE 19-5. Anatomy of the Foot. The bones of the feet, like the bones of the hand, are arranged along two arches. *From* The Columbia Presbyterian Osteoarthritis Handbook, *R. P. Grelsamer and S. Loebl, eds. Macmillan, 1996. Reproduced with permission.*

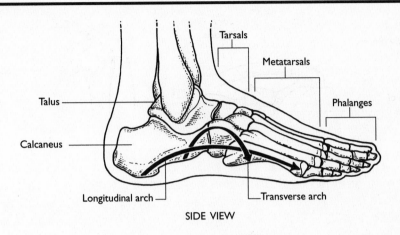

SIDE VIEW

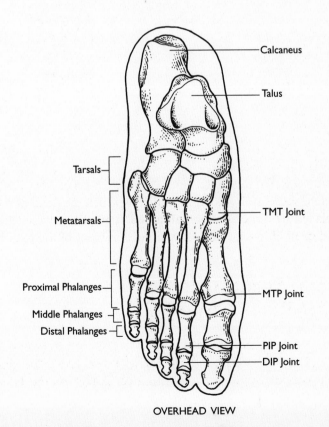

OVERHEAD VIEW

bone. The midfoot consists of five irregularly shaped bones—the *tarsals*—which, like the carpal bones of the wrist, provide a rolling motion.

The forefoot consists of five rays, ending in the toes. The long bones closest to the ankle are called the *metatarsals* (comparable to metacarpals). As with the fingers, the three following bones are called the proximal, middle, and distal phalanges (with proximal being closest to the ankle). The joints connecting these bones are called:

◆ The tarsal-metatarsal joint (TMT)

◆ The metatarsal-phalangeal joint (MTP)

◆ The proximal interphalangeal joint (PIP)

◆ The distal interphalangeal joint (DIP)

The big toe, also called the *hallux,* has only three bones instead of four. As with the hand, the bones of each foot are arranged in arches: the longitudinal arch and the transverse arch. These structures function like springs. They flatten when the foot is loaded with the weight of the body and spring back when the pressure is released.

The bones of the foot are connected with numerous ligaments. The best known of these is the Achilles tendon, which is the largest tendon of the entire body. The sole of the foot plays an important role in supporting the weight of the body and maintaining its balance. One of the layers that make up the sole is the *plantar fascia,* which runs from the heel bone and inserts itself into the nooks and crannies of the foot.

For some reason, many physicians ignore their patients' feet. Yet the feet, which bear the entire weight of the body, are extremely vulnerable and cause humanity much grief. RA often affects the numerous joints of the feet and in many patients these joints are the first target of the disease. It is crucial to stop erosion because deterioration can alter the gait pattern, which in turn stresses the knees, hips, and back. As always, RA causes inflammation and pain. Aggressive DMARD and anti-inflammatory therapy may halt joint deterioration. The importance of selecting proper shoes cannot be overemphasized (see Table 19-1).

RA often affects the MTP joint. The resulting deformation may result in *hallux valgus,* the familiar bunion characterized by the angle that forms the metatarsal and the proximal phalanx. Another common disorder is *hallux rigidus* (stiff joint of the big toe), which interferes with the smooth rolling of the foot during walking. A rheumatoid foot can develop hammer toes, resulting from inflammation of the PIP and DIP joints, and its back often widens. Other joints can become involved, deforming the foot, dislocating joints, and causing instability.

TABLE 19-1. How to Buy Properly Fitting Shoes

- Always buy your shoes in a store whose salespeople take pride in fitting you properly.
- Listen to your feet. Do not buy shoes that feel tight, loose, or cause pain or discomfort.
- Select low to average heels. 3/8 to 1 1/4 inches is good for adults.
- Be sure to select a wide, roomy toe box. Your toes should not touch the top of the shoes.
- The soles and heels should be shock-absorbing, for example, as in most sneakers and walking shoes.
- The shoes can have reinforced heels, steel shanks, arches, and/or laces.
- Shoes must fit properly. Do not try to compromise in order to save money or be in style. Most shoe stores are carpeted, and shoes that feel good in the store may pinch during normal wear. Here is what you should watch out for:

  a. Fit the shoe to both foot length and width.

  b. Use the measuring device in the shoe store. Try both the right and left shoes.

  c. Do not rely on the shoe size you have always bought. The fit may vary from style to style.

  d. Make sure that your heel fits snugly into the heel of the shoe. Watch for hard, rigid edges along the top of the shoe that may cut into your heel. Don't buy shoes that are too long or too short. Adults need an extra 3/8 to 1/2 inch from the end of the longest toe to the end of the shoe.

  e. The ball of the foot, which is the widest part of the foot, should line up with the widest part of the shoe. This fit is as important as the overall shoe length. Individuals with shortened, claw, or hammer toes should use this measure to determine the correct shoe length.

  f. The upper part of the shoe should fit comfortably over the entire foot.

  g. Buy your shoes at the end of the day when your feet are the largest.

Source: These suggestions were made by Glenn Garrison, CPO, Director of Orthotics and Prosthetics at HSS. Adapted with permission from the *Health Connection Bulletin,* volume 5, number 2.

Foot pain does not always result from arthritis. Injury of the *plantar fascia* causes pain that feels as if it were arthritis, but is not. Like RA, it is treated with rest, ice, compression (splinting), and elevation.

Initial treatment consists of anti-inflammatory drugs and a judicious mix of stress reduction, heat or cold applications, rest and activity, and cortisone injections. Stress can be reduced through use of a cane, which absorbs part of the weight that impacts during ambulation. Foot exercises are designed to maintain range of motion, maintain flexibility, and decrease pain. As always, check with your doctor before adding an exercise to your regimen.

Instead of wearing traditional shoes, some doctors recommend relying on the newer athletic footwear that reduces or eliminates the pressure exerted on the metatarsals and softens the impact during walking. Rockport shoes, with their high-wide toe box, rocker bottom, and cushioned soles, should be worn during the week and men's running shoes are recommended during the weekend. Orthotics (metatarsal pads and bars) are helpful for patients with involvement of the metatarsals.

Because feet are so exposed and delicate, foot surgery used to be considered a last resort. Today, it is often recommended in a timely fashion, before the arthritis has progressed and the dysfunctional foot has profoundly affected lifestyle. Surgery is indicated when conservative measures fail and the foot pain is constant and/or the deformities interfere with normal walking.

Podiatric surgeons commonly perform foot surgery. Two types of surgical procedures are often used: fusion (arthrodesis) and resection arthroplasty with or without surgery using implants.

During fusion, the surgeon may cut off the diseased portions of the cartilage and bones and position the cleaned ends of the tarsals in such a manner that, like the two ends of a fracture, they fuse during the healing process. Care must be taken that the bones will fuse in a useful position.

Resection arthroplasty involves the reconstruction of the entire joint. The procedure is most commonly used for correction of *hallux valgus* (bunions) but is also used for other toes.

Dr. Swanson, who developed flexible implants for the hands, developed similar devices for the feet. The purpose of these implants is to maintain the alignment of the toes, supply stability, and maintain the joint space. As for the hands, the implants are made from silicone rubber, polyethylene, and/or titanium. During resection surgery, the surgeon widens the canal of the tarsals so that the implants can be slid into place. Today, foot surgeons can select from many different implants, which differ from one another with respect to size and shape. On the average, implants last 10 to 20 years. Thereafter, a revision may become necessary.

Foot surgery used to be extremely cumbersome. The techniques, however, have improved and the procedures often do not require hospitalization. In the past, people were kept in walking casts or on crutches for months. Today, doctors may encourage weight bearing within hours after surgery. Nevertheless, the operated foot is splinted and placed in a special shoe that keeps the toes free of pressure and perfectly aligned. Full activity is usually resumed after 3 months. Foot surgery is performed under regional anesthesia (see Chapter 16).

Appendix A:
Questions and Answers
About RA

＝≈◉≈＝

Most of the material was discussed in the main portion of the *Handbook*. Some specific answers and capsule information are provided below. The questions are divided as follows:

Arthritis In General

Rheumatoid Arthritis

More About Health Care Providers

Resources

Medications

Living More Comfortably with RA

Rheumatoid Arthritis and the Work Place

Concerns After Total Joint Replacement

Alternative Therapies

ARTHRITIS IN GENERAL

What is arthritis?

Arthritis is a general term referring to any disease associated with general joint pain. Other commonly used terms include *rheumatic diseases, musculoskeletal disorders,* and *connective tissue diseases.* There are over 100 different forms of arthritis. Their common link is joint pain, but these disorders have many different causes. Osteoarthritis, which affects isolated joints, is related to degeneration of the cartilage of one or more joints. In gout, the body mishandles the breakdown of a body chemical. In infectious arthritis, bacteria attack joint tissue.

What is fibromyalgia?

Fibromyalgia is characterized by a combination of generalized and muscle pain, stiffness in and around various joints of the body, insomnia, and fatigue. The cluster of symptoms is so ill-defined that patients often have trouble obtaining a diagnosis. Unlike RA, fibromyalgia does not damage the joints. Initially, the disease may be confused with RA.

RHEUMATOID ARTHRITIS

What is rheumatoid arthritis?

In rheumatoid arthritis the immune system, whose function is to safeguard the health of the body, malfunctions and attacks its host's own tissue. This is why rheumatoid arthritis is called an *autoimmune disorder.* Initially and most markedly, this attack primarily zeroes in on the tissues found in the joints of the body, but other organs can also become involved. This is why rheumatoid arthritis is a *systemic disease* (affects the entire body.)

Who gets rheumatoid arthritis?

Most everybody can get rheumatoid arthritis, but the disease, like other autoimmune disorders, affects women disproportionately. The most common time of onset is during young and middle adulthood.

How is the disease diagnosed?

RA cannot be diagnosed by means of a single, simple laboratory test. Experienced physicians, however, can diagnose the disease quite rapidly by combining a series of tests and observations. These include:

◆ The presence of rheumatoid factor, identified by means of a laboratory test

◆ The involvement of symmetric joints (two knees, two thumbs, two hips)

◆ An elevated ESR (erythrocyte sedimentation rate) or CRP (C-reactive protein)

◆ Fatigue

Will I end up in a wheelchair?

It is unlikely that you will end up in a wheelchair. Therapy for RA has improved dramatically during the past decades. There are good drugs that will limit joint destruction. Exercise will keep your joints mobile, and surgery can repair those that are very painful or nonfunctional. However, keeping fit in spite of rheumatoid arthritis is time-consuming. Keep up the fight. It is worth it.

Can I have a baby even though I have RA?

Yes, you can have a baby even though you suffer from RA. For details, see Chapter 10.

Will my baby have RA?

No, RA is not directly inherited.

MORE ABOUT HEALTH CARE PROVIDERS

How do I locate a rheumatologist (doctor specializing in arthritis)?

◆   Ask your internist.

◆   Call the Arthritis Foundation.

◆   Most hospitals have physician referral lists. When asked, the hospital will even select physicians willing to accept a specific type of insurance.

◆   Ask a knowledgeable friend (a good way of identifying caring health care providers).

◆   Call your local medical society.

Once you have obtained one or more names, you may wish to read up on the physician in *The Official ABMS Directory of Board Certified Medical Specialists*. The book is available at most libraries. This information can also be obtained on the Web: www.ABMS.org.

How do I locate other health care providers?

Your rheumatologist, internist, or primary care physician will be able to put you in touch with physical therapists and surgeons. Also, use the sources mentioned above.

What is an osteopath?

Osteopathy is a system of medicine founded in the United States in 1874 by Dr. Andrew Taylor Still. Osteopaths believe that disease results from the disturbance (malfunction) of a particular part of the body, which then affects overall function. Treatment is aimed at reestablishing this balance by conventional medical methods involving drugs, surgery, and physical manipulation. Osteopathic physicians (D.O.) are full-fledged members of the medical community, with all the rights and obligations this entails.

What is a chiropractor?

A chiropractor believes that diseases, especially those related to the back, are associated with an abnormal function of the spinal system. Symptoms may be relieved by an appropriate manipulation of the spine.

What is a podiatrist?

Podiatrists specialize in the treatment and care of the feet and play an important role in any disease in which walking may be difficult. Podiatrists help you to maintain optimal use of your feet. They do such mundane tasks as cutting toenails. They provide useful advice about buying shoes. They also prescribe and make inlays. Podiatrists are licensed to prescribe medications and to perform foot surgery.

RESOURCES

Where can I get reliable information about RA?

The Arthritis Foundation (AF) is a voluntary health agency dealing with all forms of arthritis. It is located at 1330 West Peachtree St., Atlanta, GA 30309. It has a national toll-free telephone number (800–283–7800) staffed by volunteers who provide information about arthritis in general and RA in particular. The foundation publishes a series of free booklets dealing with the various forms of arthritis, as well as with specific issues such as fatigue, activities, pain, stress reduction, tips on traveling with arthritis, and other topics. The foundation has a Web site at www.arthritis.org that provides information on some new drugs and other developments. The site provides numerous links to other Web sites and chat rooms dealing with RA. Caution is recommended. Just because information is on the Web does not make it reliable. The Arthritis Foundation has about 70 chapters throughout the United States. You can join AF for a small annual fee and receive their excellent magazine called *Arthritis Today*.

In Canada, information is provided by The Arthritis Society (TAS) at 250 Bloor St. East, Suite 901, Toronto, Ontario M4W 3P2 (800–321–1433). The society has links to a network of provincial divisions. It also has a very informative Web site, www.arthritis.ca, and a magazine.

The American College of Rheumatology has a large website at www. rheumatology.org that provides information on many relevant aspects of your care (specific disease, drugs, advances in research). The Web site is cross-linked to others that offer alternative care. Read the information critically, because it may not necessarily be accurate.

The public library is also an excellent source for reliable information. Look for general books about arthritis and those that discuss rheumatoid arthritis. Medical encyclopedias such as those put out by Columbia Presbyterian Medical Center (now New York–Presbyterian), the Mayo Clinic, and the American Medical Association are also helpful. You can read up on your prescription drugs in the *Physicians' Desk Reference. Infomedicine: A Consumer's Guide to the Latest Medical Research* provides what its title indicates. The *Reader's Guide to Periodic Literature* indexes articles on specific subjects that have appeared in consumer magazines.

More information is available in medical libraries. Discuss possible access with your local librarian. In a medical library you may tackle medical textbooks and specialty journals (*Arthritis and Rheumatism, Journal of Rheumatology, Arthritis Care and Research*). These may be difficult to read, and you may need a medical dictionary to help you understand certain medical terms. You can look up abstracts of articles in the *Index Medicus,* available in medical libraries. This mammoth compendium is the professional equivalent of the *Guide to Periodic Literature*. It abstracts articles from 4,000 medical journals.

My health insurance denied my claim. What should I do?

The problem is so widespread that several newly formed organizations now deal with it. As of this writing, two professionals who deal with specific problems were identified. They are Roland Cassavant, a certified claims assistant professional (800–556–7117; www.consumermedhelp.com), and Susan Dressler (877–275–8765; www.claims.org).

In telephone interviews both seemed knowledgeable. They will handle problems with medication reimbursement, surgery, home health care, and so on. Cassavant, who charges $1.99 per minute on the telephone, says that consultations usually last 20 minutes. Sometimes he tells clients of alternate ways of handling problems. Dressler formed a voluntary health agency called the Alliance of Claims Assistant Professionals (ACAP), an umbrella for 85 professionals throughout the United States. Her members charge between $20 and $60 an hour to provide advice, make phone calls, write letters, and fill out claim forms. ACAP also negotiates fee reduction for portions of the bill not covered by insurance.

MEDICATIONS

What medications are used to treat RA?

About 50 different medications are used to treat RA. These are discussed in detail in Chapters 6 through 9.

What are monoclonal antibodies?

These substances are chemically and immunologically pure antibodies produced by cells in a test tube. They are aimed at specific portions of proteins and can be used diagnostically to identify specific diseases and therapeutically to treat tumors and arthritis.

Why are there so many different drugs to treat RA?

First, many of the medications used to treat arthritis have been developed during the past 50 years as our understanding of RA and of drug technology has improved. Second, the immune and inflammatory systems of the body are quite complex. The optimal suppression and resetting of the abnormalities found in RA necessitate an array of medications, each focused at a different site. Furthermore, the body chemistry of different patients varies greatly. Therefore, each person needs his or her individually crafted drug regimen.

What is the difference between the various NSAIDs?

While many of these nonsteroidal anti-inflammatory drugs are variations on a similar chemical theme, they differ sufficiently in their basic structure to affect patients differently with regard to clinical improvement and side effects. One patient may fail on one drug or have major stomach irritation with one NSAID and have a superb reduction in joint inflammation and no side effects with another. Because building an appropriate blood level with one drug may take up to 3 weeks, your doctor will try one NSAID for 3 to 4 weeks. If you do not respond or if you have side effects, he or she will stop the first drug and begin a second NSAID and observe your response. This type of trial and error is quite usual and unfortunately there is no way to predict which one of these medications will lead to a clinical improvement without having side effects.

How long should I try a particular DMARD before giving up?

Disease-modifying antirheumatic drugs differ greatly in their personality. They also have separate timelines with regard to clinical response. A response with

Plaquenil and sulfasalazine takes 3 to 4 months to manifest itself. During this time, NSAIDs and a short course of steroids can be used as a bridge until improvement becomes noticeable. Methotrexate works a bit faster. Improvements are noted after 4 to 6 weeks. Often, the initial dose has to be increased to 20 to 25 mg/week before a noticeable response occurs, again increasing the time it takes to evaluate a new drug. Enbrel commonly works quickly, within 2 to 3 weeks.

Why do corticosteroids have to be discontinued so slowly?

When patients take steroids for more than a month, their own adrenal gland production of steroids is curtailed. Thus, when you decrease your dose of steroids, it needs to be done slowly, because your body has to adjust to the lower dose. It takes 9 to 12 months for your adrenal glands to resume their steroid production.

What is the difference between Enbrel and Remicade?

Both drugs interfere with the tumor necrosis factor-alpha (TNF-a), a particular cytokine (body chemical) produced by the immune system that is believed to play a crucial role in initiating the chronic joint inflammation characteristic of rheumatoid arthritis. Use of the TNF-alpha inhibitors in the treatment of RA started in 1999. Initial results are extremely promising. Enbrel provides a fake receptor for TNF-alpha. Remicade blocks the body's own receptor. Either way, the effects of TNF-alpha are not transmitted.

Currently, there is no information as to which one of the two drugs is better. As with many other medications, the answer will come from long-term trials.

What is all that fuss about that super-aspirin (COX-2 inhibitors)?

One family of chemicals the body uses to run itself is the prostaglandins. All prostaglandins originate in the cell membrane, and then differentiate. Each one of these slightly different prostaglandins has a job. Some participate in producing mucus that protects the lining of the stomach. Others regulate kidney function, blood pressure, inflammation, and pain. Aspirin, the NSAIDs, and the new COX-2 inhibitors interfere with prostaglandin production. Aspirin, however, blocks prostaglandin production early in the game, thereby doing away with a good prostaglandin that is involved in coating the stomach. The COX-2 inhibitors swing into action later, permitting the production of good prostaglandins and selectively interfering with those that cause pain and inflammation.

LIVING MORE COMFORTABLY WITH RA

Is there a way to shorten morning stiffness?

Many patients figure out how to shorten their morning stiffness. Here are suggestions that may work:

- Start your day with a hot bath or shower.
- Take medication in the evening, which still has some beneficial effects in the morning.
- Stretch before getting out of bed.
- Warm your clothes in the dryer before putting them on.

Should I move to Florida or Arizona since I feel worse in cold, clammy weather?

The change to a warm climate helps for only a short while. Then the body adjusts and the disease returns. Since a warm, dry climate will not alter your RA, you should not move away from family and friends just because of your disease. You may, however, profit from taking a warm-weather vacation in winter.

How can I be less tired?

Chronic fatigue is one of the most unpleasant aspects of RA. You will be less tired once your symptoms are adequately controlled by DMARDs. However, it is important to remember that you should not overtax yourself. RA affects your entire body. If you can, rest during the day. Ask others to relieve you of as much physical work as possible. Do not waste your strength on shopping, cleaning, and carrying heavy items.

RA AND THE WORK PLACE

What should I tell my boss about my RA?

Most people are conflicted about talking about their disease at work. Unfortunately, there are no clear guidelines, and each patient is on his or her own. Informing supervisors and colleagues about suffering from a chronic disease may stigmatize you as a victim. In extreme cases, a chronic disease characterized by pain and fatigue may arouse suspicion of malingering. Though it should not, the knowledge that an employee has a chronic health problem may interfere with promotions and choice assignments.

On the other hand, not talking about a disease as disabling as RA is extremely stressful. Moreover, it may make it more difficult to work less during a flare, get time off for doctors' appointments, or obtain special equipment or a reduced workweek. A track record of having a chronic illness is also important if you have to apply for disability.

The Americans with Disability Act (ADA), passed in 1990, obviously covers people suffering from RA. The act also obliges employers to help the disabled to continue working by providing them with adaptive equipment. Extensive information about the ADA can be found on the Web at www.usdoj.gov/crt/ada/pubs or by calling 800–514–0301.

According to Susan Milstrey Wells, author of *A Delicate Balance: Living Successfully with Chronic Illness* (Insight Books/Plenum Press, 1998), most people have to apply repeatedly before disability is granted.

CONCERNS AFTER TOTAL JOINT REPLACEMENT

What about going to the dentist after joint replacement?

You must inform your dentist of the fact that you had a total joint replacement. Very rarely, dental work may cause late joint infection, which in turn may cause loosening of the artificial joint, especially if it is weight bearing (hips or knees). You may be instructed to take an antibiotic 1 or 2 hours before your appointment and another dose later that day. The need for this precaution is controversial. Nevertheless, it is advisable to provide the dentist with your complete medical history. Also inform your dentist of drug allergies.

What about diagnostic tests after joint replacement?

You may be advised to take antibiotics before an invasive test such as a cystoscopy. In any case, you should inform all your doctors of your artificial joint(s) in order to avoid accidental dislocation during, for example, a gynecological examination.

ALTERNATIVE THERAPIES

Should I try bee stings?

During the past decades, it has been reported that bee venom relieves the pain and inflammation of RA. The reports have been so consistent that they have been investigated by a number of top-notch arthritis investigators. There is still no definite answer as to whether apitherapy (medical use of bee products) is successful. According to Dr. Robert Zurier, director of rheumatology at the Massachusetts Medical School, bee venom may work, but he does not use it because he has so many better, less painful ways to treat RA. In addition to pain, bee venom may cause a severe allergic reaction.

What about glucosamine and chondroitin sulfate?

Since 1997, it has been reported that glucosamine and condroitin sulfate supplements will cure arthritis. Patients have been flocking to health food stores to buy the supplements. Both glucosamine and condroitin sulfate are natural substances that are part of cartilage. There is no evidence that these substances are absorbed into cartilage when taken by mouth.

Since so many people report feeling better when they take the supplements, scientists have been trying to figure out the reason. Speculation about the beneficial effects of chondroitin sulfate and glucosamine include:

♦ The substances act as a mild analgesic (painkiller).

♦ People taking glucosamine and condroitin sulfate are advised to exercise and diet while taking the supplements. The overall therapy might be beneficial.

♦ The substances may inhibit some of the enzymes involved with cartilage degradation.

♦ Most of us feel better when we do something about whatever disease we are suffering from. Since arthritis in general, and RA in particular, varies from day to day, this so-called placebo effect is particularly marked.

For more information, see Judith Horstman, *The Arthritis Foundation's Guide to Alternative Therapies*. Arthritis Foundation. Atlanta, Georgia, 1999.

Appendix B: Glossary[1]

analgesia, analgesic   *Algos* is pain in Greek. Combined with *an* ("no"), it means "no pain." The term most commonly refers to medications that eliminate pain.

antibodies   Special proteins generated by the body in response to an infectious agent or other foreign substance.

antigen   A substance the immune system considers "foreign" and/or "nonself" and against which it mounts an immune response.

arthritis   A general term referring to inflammation of the joints

arthrodesis   Refers to fusion of two bones.

arthroscope   A fiber-optic instrument that permits physicians to look into the joints and perform minor surgical repairs.

autoantibodies   Antibody that form against a person's own tissues.

B cells   A subgroup of lymphocytes, which, among other functions, manufacture antibodies.

Bouchard's node   Bony enlargements forming on the proximal joints of the fingers. This growth is characteristic of osteoarthritis and not RA.

---

[1]Some of these definitions were adapted from the Rheumatoid Arthritis: Information Package, prepared by National Institutes of Arthritis, Musculoskeletal and Skin Diseases (NIAMSD).

cartilage   The tough, elastic tissue that covers and cushions the ends of the bones and absorbs shock.

collagen   The principal structural protein of the body encountered in skin, bone, tendons, ligaments, cartilage, and connective tissues.

connective tissue   A general term referring to the tissues that support the body and its internal organs.

C-reactive protein   A specific protein produced during inflammation. It is elevated in RA and used to gauge the activity of the disease.

cytokines   A group of body chemicals that participate in inflammation.

diarthroidal joint   A joint that allows free movement in one or more directions. The joints of the fingers, hands, elbows, knees, and hips are good examples. RA can affect most diarthroidal joints.

DMARD   Short for disease-modifying antirheumatic drug, such as methotrexate, gold, and antimalarials.

erosion   In our context, refers to the wearing or destruction of joint surfaces as a consequence of the inflammatory processes characteristic of RA.

erythrocyte sedimentation rate (ESR)   The rate at which red blood cells settle in a test tube. An elevated ESR is a sign of inflammation. The ESR is elevated in RA and the degree of elevation is a sign of the severity of the disease.

exercise, active   Unassisted exercises as when you bend and extend a leg.

exercise, isometric   Tightening of muscles without moving the joint.

exercise, isotonic   Moving a joint through its partial or entire range of motion.

exercise, passive   A physical therapist moves the joint through its range of motion.

extension   Straightening of a joint.

extra-articular   Literally means "outside the joint." In our context, refers to manifestations such as anemia, ulcers, or Felty's syndrome that may accompany RA.

fibrous capsule   The tough envelope of tendons and ligaments surrounding a joint.

flare   Sudden worsening of symptoms in RA.

flexion   Bending of a joint.

flexion contracture   The shrinking or narrowing that occurs when the joint loses some or all of its range of motion. When extreme, flexion contractures can lead to the complete loss of function of a joint.

genetic marker   A particular hereditary gene or set of genes that increase the risk of developing a particular disease. Certain forms of arthritis, especially ankylosing spondylitis, are associated with such a genetic marker.

Heberden's node   Bony enlargement seen on the distal interphalangeal joint. This growth is characteristic of osteoarthritis and not RA.

immune modulators   Refers to substances that affect and/or modify the immune response. Currently, the term refers to medications such as Enbrel (etanercept) that specifically interfere with the immune response.

immunosuppressant   A drug that depresses the immune system.

inflammation   A characteristic response of tissue to injury or disease. Its four classic manifestations include swelling, redness, warmth, and pain.

joint capsule   See *fibrous capsule*.

joint space   The space between the ends of the bones in a joint that allows for effortless motion. Inflammation reduces the joint space, and loss of joint space is an early symptom of arthritis.

lymphocytes   A specific group of white blood cells that play a crucial role in the inflammation characteristic of RA.

nonsteroidal anti-inflammatory drugs (NSAIDs)   Drugs such as aspirin that moderate and/or suppress inflammation (anti-inflammatory) but are not steroids such as prednisone.

osteoblasts   Specialized cells that form new bone.

osteoclasts   Specialized cells that remove bone.

osteophytes   Bone spurs.

pannus   A pile-up of inflammatory cells and debris developing in the joint as a consequence of inflammation.

prostaglandins   Hormone-like substances originating in the cell membrane that regulate many physiological processes including kidney function, blood pressure, secretion of the mucus coating the stomach, and inflammation.

range of motion (ROM)   A measurement of the ability of the joint to go through all its normal motions.

rectal   Medication prepared as suppositories so that it can be administered in the anus.

remission   A state during which the symptoms of the disease are lessened or absent. A marked decrease in the duration of morning stiffness is one symptom of remission.

rheumatoid factor   An abnormal antibody found in 80 percent of those suffering from RA.

sedimentation rate   The speed at which the red blood cells settle in a calibrated tube. An increased rate is indicative of inflammation.

suspension   A drug dispersed in liquid form.

synovial fluid   A viscous fluid produced by the synovium, which nourishes and lubricates the joint.

synovium   The cellophane-like tissue that lines the joint capsule. The synovium produces the synovial fluid, which lubricates the joint. In RA, the thin synovium becomes inflamed and swells.

systemic   Affecting the entire body.

T cells   A subgroup of lymphocytes especially involved in the inflammation characteristic of RA.

TNF-alpha   Abbreviation for tumor necrosis factor-alpha. TNF-alpha is one of many cytokines. It, however, plays a major role in fueling the self-perpetuating inflammatory response characteristic of RA. The new immunomodulator drugs (Remicade and Inflimax) block TNF-alpha from reaching their receptors, thereby interrupting the inflammatory processes.

Index